The *Crowood Health Guides* are designed to offer practical
guidance in coping with common health problems. Each title is
written by an experienced practitioner within the specific field,
and each aims at providing a clear, reliable and responsible
introduction for those concerned, their families and those who
care for them. Adopting a readable style and with clear line
illustration, the series is a major contribution to the growing
health debate and puts much-needed information in the hands of
those directly involved.

Arthritis

A Practical Guide to Coping

Dr Richard Price

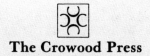

The Crowood Press

First published in 1988 by
The Crowood Press
Ramsbury, Marlborough,
Wiltshire SN8 2HE

British Library Cataloguing in Publication Data

Price, Richard
Arthritis.
1. Man. Joints. Arthritis
I. Title
616.7'22

ISBN 1 85223 064 9

Acknowledgements

Many thanks to Jane Williams for her skilled and patient help
with the preparation of the manuscript.

Picture Credits

Line illustrations by Claire Upsdale-Jones

Typeset by Avonset, Midsomer Norton, Bath
Printed in Great Britain at The Bath Press

Contents

Preface

Pain in the muscles, joints and related structures is one of the commonest reasons for seeing the doctor. Much of it is due to non-serious conditions which will clear up spontaneously or with simple treatment. However, such is the widespread ignorance about arthritic conditions that sufferers are frequently over-anxious, feeling that they have a relentless, crippling disease and simultaneously thinking that 'nothing can be done'. Ignorance is not meant to be a disparaging term: it means lack of knowledge, not stupidity, and is also widespread among doctors. This arises because rheumatology, that branch of medicine concerned with the non-surgical study of conditions, is relatively new. It is worth recalling that its growth to become a major subspeciality of medicine has coincided with the provision of the National Health Service in Great Britain. This allows for the treatment of long-standing conditions which private health systems can rarely afford to cover adequately and elsewhere, in practice, do not.

It is the purpose of this book to provide for patients basic, orthodox information and explanations about the rheumatic diseases. It is not an aid to self-diagnosis and I assume that you will consult your own doctor. It is intended, rather, to clarify and amplify information which may not have been taken in (or given) at a busy and unnerving clinic attendance. I believe that if patients understand their illness they are less 'dis-abled' by it, and if they understand how their doctors think they can get more out of them and establish a better, trusting relationship that is the key to all medical practice.

Dr Richard Price
October 1987

1
What is Arthritis?

INTRODUCTION

The words arthritis and rheumatism cause a lot of confusion. This is increased by their combined use in the term rheumatoid arthritis. Since many assume that all arthritis implies an inevitably crippling, untreatable condition, the diagnosis causes much anxiety.

The ending '—itis' implies inflammation, hence appendicitis, and so from the Greek '*arthros*', meaning a joint, we get arthritis – inflammation of a joint. The nature of inflammation is discussed later in this chapter. However, since all arthritis may not be inflammatory, some doctors have preferred words such as arthropathy – disease of joints (compare psychopathy, disease of the psyche, or personality) – and arthrosis, which has a similar meaning (compare psychosis). But the term arthritis has stuck through common use and implies a disease which damages the moving surfaces of joints, usually causing the joint to become swollen.

Rheumatism is a word that has no specific meaning and is used more by patients than doctors. It has origins in the old medical concept of 'rheum' meaning watery secretions and relating to diseases caused by damp conditions. Nowadays doctors use it to refer to any aches and pains in the muscles, bones or joints for which they have no explanation and, most importantly, which they consider non-serious. Specialist rheumatologists like to use the word in a more limited sense, as in 'soft-tissue rheumatism', meaning identifiable but non-arthritic conditions, usually of muscles, ligaments and tendons.

Unfortunately, the prefix 'rheum' is also used in three specific diseases, rheumatoid arthritis, polymyalgia rheumatica and rheumatic fever, which is rather confusing. Its use in these terms reflects the fact that general stiffness and aching are a major feature of these illnesses, in addition to simple pain.

Although 'arthritis' has a specific meaning, it is not a single disease. Most people are unaware that there are about 200 different types of arthritis, often widely different and varying from trivial to severe. Some arthritic conditions do not confine their attack to the joints but give rise to general disease affecting other organs as well. Consequently, information you may hear about a friend's illness may not apply to your own, causing unnecessary worry and perhaps inappropriate treatment.

JOINT STRUCTURE

A joint is a connection between bones. Arthritic conditions mainly affect the moving joints, called synovial joints (*see* Fig 1). The joints in your thumb are simple examples of such joints – the moving surfaces of the bone are lined with smooth cartilage, which is the pearly gristle you see on a pig's trotter in the butcher's shop. The easy movement of the joint is lubricated by a thin film of synovial fluid made by cells of the joint lining, or synovium, and this fluid also provides nutrients for the cartilage. Outside the synovium is the tough fibrous joint capsule containing nerve endings which can signal pain.

Although the basic processes vary in different arthritic diseases, they often include inflammation and swelling of the synovial lining, with increased fluid production leading to a swollen joint. There

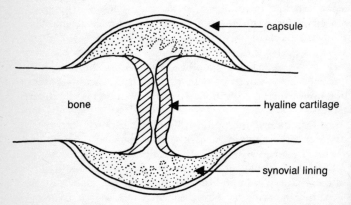

Fig 1   A section through a typical synovial joint.

may also be destruction of cartilage and ultimately, in severe cases, wear of the underlying bone. The capsule of many joints is reinforced in places by thickened bands of fibrous tissue called ligaments, which restrict movement of the joint in certain directions and so increase its stability. When a joint becomes swollen these ligaments become stretched so that the joint becomes wobbly.

Joints are moved by muscles, attached to the bone or capsule alongside the joint by condensed, rope-like masses of fibrous tissue called tendons. To allow free play of the tendons as their muscles contract they run in close-fitting fibrous sheaths, separated by a film of lubricating fluid. The lining of these sheaths and the fluid they produce are much the same as that of the synovial cells and joint fluid so, not surprisingly, inflammation of tendons is a feature of many arthritic conditions.

In certain regions, friction between groups of tendons, muscle and nearby structures is prevented by a larger pouch of fluid called a bursa. Inflammation of a bursa is a bursitis and since many bursae lie adjacent to joints, bursitis sometimes mimics arthritis, although it is not serious and is easily treated.

CONNECTIVE TISSUE

The whole of the body is made up of microscopic living units called cells. Each cell contains a nucleus carrying inherited genes in the form of a chemical code which has the information to make all the components of that individual. The rest of the cell is a chemical factory turning these genetic plans into working molecules, whether structural materials or enzymes which run the chemical reactions that make us alive. The cells lie in an immediate environment of watery or semi-solid matter of their own making – the ground substance. During development cells come to only a part of their genetic potential and so become specialised. Aggregations of similarly specialised cells, their ground substance and the products they secrete into it constitute the different tissues of the body.

Musculo-skeletal structures are all modifications of a single tissue type, connective tissue. Simple, loose forms of this tissue constitute the packing within and between organs and contain a number of cell types: fibroblasts, which make tough, fibrous material called collagen, and macrophages and mast cells, which have a major role in initiating and orchestrating inflammatory responses to injury. At such times the cell complement of connective tissue is increased by the migration of cells from the blood.

Ligaments and tendons are connective tissues almost entirely comprising the collagen fibre elements, while muscle consists in large part of cells packed with contractile protein. Bone is specialised by the formation of material containing calcium in the ground substance, but there are also, nevertheless, many fibres in bone, to give tensile strength. The cells are modified either to make bone (osteoblasts) or to dissolve and remodel it (osteoclasts). The ground substance of the glassy cartilage lining the joint is thickened to a jelly-like consistency by the addition of very large organic molecules (proteoglycans) which retain water, so giving the tissue shock-absorbing properties. The cartilage cells, unlike bone, do not regenerate, so damage tends to be additive. About a third of the cells of the synovial lining of the joint are rather like fibroblasts and contribute to the chemical contents of synovial fluid, but the rest are mostly macrophages. Since synovium is also very vascular, the scope for immunologically mediated inflammation in joints is considerable.

INFLAMMATION AND THE IMMUNE SYSTEM

The immune system is the means by which living things detect the intrusion of foreign material, for example, viruses, and mobilise tissue responses to such injury, of which the most central is the range of co-ordinated reactions we call inflammation. It is certain that much of the pain and damage of arthritis, as in other diseases, is a consequence of inflammatory activity and there is increasing belief that many arthritic conditions begin as disorders of the immune process, due in part to genetic variation in the immune system between individuals.

We are all familiar with inflammation in the form of a mosquito bite or a boil and its features were recognised and listed centuries ago as heat (*calor*), redness (*rubor*), swelling (*turgor*), and pain (*dolor*), all leading to loss of function of the affected part. Subsequent science has shown that these outward signs have their basis in the dilatation of local blood vessels under the influence of mediator substances released in damaged tissue (for example, from mast cells). These blood vessels become more permeable and more cells and activating chemicals migrate from the blood into the tissues, sustaining and extending the inflammatory mechanisms by which invading organisms may be destroyed. The cells include certain white blood cells called polymorphs which release enzymes capable of digesting the tissue of host and invader alike. Vast aggregations of these white cells form the material we call pus.

More macrophages are added to those already present in the tissues and contribute additional chemical mediators capable of activating or suppressing other cells and initiating cell destroying processes. One such substance is Interleukin I which probably plays a large part in generating the general symptoms of inflammatory illnesses such as fever, feeling rotten and loss of appetite and weight. Macrophages (literally 'big eaters') ingest debris and alert other cells of the immune system – the B lymphocytes – to recognise part of the chemical structure of the invading virus or bacterium as foreign (the antigen). In turn, the B lymphocytes construct more or less specific proteins (antibodies) which then attach to identical antigens on still-living invader organisms and help destroy them. These antibodies can be detected in the blood and can be used in the diagnosis of present and past infection.

The production of antibodies by B cells after macrophage activation requires the additional help of a different class of lymphocytes, the T cells. Not all T cells are helpers; another group have a suppressing effect on the immune process and it is interesting that the ratio of T-helper to T-suppressor cells varies from normal in some arthritic conditions. A further class of T cells responds directly to antigens presented by macrophages. It transforms into cells capable of killing foreign cells carrying that antigen (cell-mediated immunity) or releases active mediator substances such as Interferon which prevents the replication of viruses and which has begun to be used in the treatment of some diseases.

The attachment of killer cell or antibody to the antigen triggers many of the non-specific but highly toxic forces of inflammation and, in addition, can set off chemical chain reactions in the blood (cascade reactions) which widen the inflammatory response even further, rather like a guided missile hitting a petrol store.

While this warfare is taking place with its inevitable innocent casualties among the body's own tissues, normal tissue components such as fibroblasts begin to repair the damage. In some organs repair is limited to an infill of collagen fibres (scar tissue), in others the specialised working cells of the tissue can regenerate and resume normal function.

In the case of the arthritic disease it is easy to see the destructive potential of an inflammatory response occurring in a joint invaded by a bacterial infection (that is, a septic arthritis) but in other conditions, such as rheumatoid arthritis there is no obvious foreign cause for the inflammation in the joints. We therefore have to imagine that the immune system is haywire. It either wrongly identifies normal tissue as foreign (auto-immunity), or continues, inappropriately, to fight age-old battles against previous infections because it cannot fully overcome them or because it cannot switch off the immune response. Such abnormalities may represent genetic flaws in the immune system. There is support for such ideas in several arthritic diseases.

The chemical structure of the proteins on the cell surface of lymphocytes and macrophages that allow them to recognise each other and co-operate in making antibodies and killer cells depends on genes of the HLA system (Human Leucocyte (white cell) Antigen system). Genetic variations in HLA genes between individuals could therefore lead to deficiencies or quirks in the immune system which might allow an inappropriate inflammatory response to arise, or to persist, and result in an inflammatory disease. Very many associations are now known between the inheritance of a particular HLA pattern and a tendency to particular diseases, including arthritic ones. These connections are, however, nearly all fairly loose, suggesting that for diseases to develop, the genetically predisposed individual needs to meet an environmental factor (a virus maybe?). Such ideas lie behind much modern research in rheumatology.

2
Soft Tissue Rheumatism

Soft tissue rheumatism represents a range of localised, painful conditions of muscles, tendons, ligaments, etc., where the joints themselves are not involved. Although these conditions are incredibly common, they are often poorly recognised by non-specialists and can give rise to disproportionate anxiety that the patient has a serious arthritis which may spread. In fact, they nearly always clear up on their own or respond well to simple treatment.

Sometimes the cause of the condition is obvious – an injury, or repetitive wear, for example – and some forms occur, although rarely, as part of another disease. A few types of soft tissue rheumatism are more common in people who also have a true arthritis but the vast majority of cases represent just one of those things sent to try us and will get better.

FORMS OF SOFT TISSUE RHEUMATISM

Nerve Entrapment

This arises when a nerve passes through a confined space between tough structures such as ligaments and bones. Mostly it occurs for no clear reason, but obviously it is more likely to develop if the local anatomy becomes distorted and narrows the gap still further.

If you develop a nerve entrapment you might notice pain in the region supplied by the nerve, or altered sensations such as a feeling of 'pins and needles', or numbness such as after a dental anaesthetic. There may be weakness and later loss of muscle bulk (wasting).

Carpal Tunnel Syndrome

This is the best-known nerve entrapment involving the median nerve as it passes across the wrist to supply thumb muscles and

13

sensation to the thumb and first three fingers. At the wrist (*carpus* in Latin) it runs between the small wrist bones and a transverse fibrous ligament (*see* Fig 2), competing for space in this tunnel with tendons passing to the fingers.

The nerve may be trapped in rheumatoid arthritis when there is a swelling of the tendons and the wrist joint. The condition also occurs in women who are pregnant, using oral contraceptives or at the menopause, times when hormonal changes cause generalised soft tissue swelling. Deposits of amorphous material in the tunnel may explain carpal tunnel syndrome in diabetes or when the thyroid gland is underactive. In most cases the patient is otherwise healthy but experiences pain, numbness, clumsiness or weakness of the hand, especially in the early hours of the morning. Sometimes the pain spreads right up the arm. Shaking the hand or dangling it out of bed may bring relief. The doctor may be able to detect that the nerve is trapped by examination, but often he is sure on the story alone. If there is doubt he may arrange an EMG (electromyogram) which detects where nerve activity is slowed.

Treatment may include a light wrist splint or an attempt to 'dry out' the tissues with a diuretic (water tablet) which increases salt

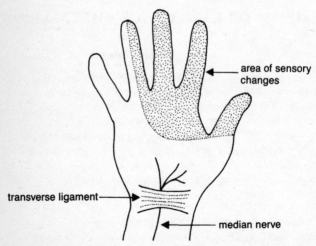

area of sensory changes

transverse ligament

median nerve

Fig 2   Carpal tunnel syndrome.

and water loss in the urine. More usual, and better, is an injection of a little steroid into the tunnel which quickly reduces swelling and frees the nerve. If the problem recurs frequently, or if muscle weakness is present, the doctor will recommend a simple operation to divide the transverse ligament. Surgeons usually prefer you to have a general anaesthetic but it is often done as a day case.

Ulnar Nerve Entrapment

The ulnar is an important nerve running behind the inner side of the elbow in a bony groove to supply vital hand muscles and sensation to the ring and little fingers (*see* Fig 3). A blow on this nerve gives rise to that awful tingling pain you get when you 'hit your funny bone'. The nerve may become damaged at the elbow and it is so important that surgery is usually advised to move the nerve in front of the joint where it does not get stretched so much.

Tarsal Tunnel Syndrome

The tibial nerve may be trapped as it passes through the tarsal tunnel in the ankle giving burning pain in the sole. It is a lot less common than carpal tunnel syndrome but may also be found in

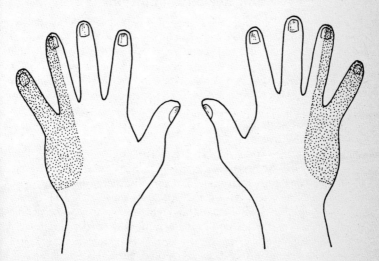

Fig 3   Sensory changes in ulnar nerve entrapment.

rheumatoid arthritis. Rheumatoid patients with new pains in the hands or feet should not assume they are due to worsening of their joints but report them to their doctor because relief of nerve entrapment can give dramatic improvement.

Meralgia Paraesthetica

This is a numb, painful sensation in front of the thigh due to trapping of an unimportant sensory nerve in the groin. It can be injected or released but does not usually need treatment. It may be mistaken for more important conditions such as arthritis of the hip.

Common Peroneal Entrapment

The nerve runs around the outer side of the knee and pressure on it while sitting cross-legged causes 'pins and needles'. In some bedridden patients blankets may press on it long enough to paralyse the foot muscles so that the foot droops and this may take weeks to recover.

Tennis Elbow, Golfer's Elbow and Related Conditions

At its lower end, the upper arm bone (humerus) widens to form two prominences which you can feel at either side of the elbow. At the outer of these are the fibrous attachments of the muscles which extend the wrist and fingers and are used whenever you lift, push or carry a heavy object. Tennis elbow arises when some of these fibres tear away from the bone and it can be excruciating. Obviously, the extensor muscles are going to be stressed in many situations other than tennis and most sufferers have never lifted a racket in their lives.

The symptoms are of pain and tenderness at the outer side of the elbow. Forcing the muscles, by carrying a heavy case, for example, increases the pain which may then spread up and down the arm. Left alone, and especially if the damaged muscle can be rested, most tennis elbows will heal within eighteen months. Some people find that thickening the handle of any implement they use regularly will reduce pain on gripping. In light occupations a wrist splint may limit extensor muscle activity and cure the tennis elbow. However, the usual treatment is a steroid injection into the tender area. In the rare circumstances of frequent recurrence, an operation may be offered to separate and reattach the torn muscle.

Golfer's elbow is the same problem at the inner aspect of the elbow affecting the flexor muscles. It is usually less troublesome and, again, most patients do not play golf.

Achilles tendonitis affects the attachment of the Achilles tendon to the back of the heel.

Plantar fasciitis is a similar inflammatory condition under the heel at the attachment of the broad fibrous band which runs forward under the foot to support the arch.

All these conditions produce local pain and tenderness and are treated by local steroid injections or soft padding. Even stubborn cases get better eventually.

Tendonitis

Inflammation of a tendon or its sheath (tendonitis or tenosynovitis) causes swelling and prevents movement of related joints because tendon contraction is painful. Tendonitis of the fingers causes them to be swollen like bananas and can be an early feature of some true arthritic conditions. The patient cannot 'make a fist'.

Trigger Finger or Thumb

Inflammation of the flexor tendon to finger or thumb may result in a localised swelling which can be felt. When the finger is bent the muscle can pull the nodule through the narrow tendon sheath but when the finger tries to straighten, a weaker action, the nodule sticks in the sheath and the finger remains bent. It can be freed by forcing it with the other hand when it suddenly straightens with a click. This is quite common in otherwise normal people and can be treated by injection of steroid into the sheath or by splitting the sheath surgically.

Tendon Rupture

When tendons are severely inflamed, as in rheumatoid arthritis, they may rupture (snap). This is more serious and, where possible, early attempts are made to repair them.

De Quervain's Tenosynovitis

This is inflammation of tendons passing across the base of the thumb which are often visibly swollen and tender if stretched by forcibly bending the thumb. Traditionally, the patient feels pain lifting a teapot. Injection therapy is very effective.

Ganglia

Ganglia are fluid-filled swellings along the line of a tendon sheath and are harmless. Steroid injections shrink them but some patients want them surgically removed. Traditionally they were dispersed by a blow from the family Bible, but the ideological content is not important since *Das Kapital* is just as effective.

Knee and Ankle Ligaments

At each side of the knee and the ankle are strong ligaments which prevent sideways dislocation of the joint. Twisting injuries commonly strain or tear them, causing exquisite tenderness to pressure or stretching of the ligament. Although these injuries always heal they may take many months, so that patients often lose confidence in their doctor's reassurances and 'want something to be done'. There is, in fact, little to be done except to use support strapping and, in the case of nasty ankle strains, physiotherapy with a balance board which trains the muscles around the joint to provide additional support may be helpful. Strengthening the thigh muscles (quadriceps) similarly helps the strained knee.

Tears of the Knee Cartilage

Everyone has heard of sportsmen having a cartilage operation. The cartilage in question is not the smooth lining surface of the joint, but two crescent-shaped pads made of cartilage, reinforced by criss-crossed fibrous tissue designed to spread the weight of the body from femur to tibia.

A torn cartilage typically follows a twisting injury and occurs in non-athletic people too. There is immediate pain and soon the knee becomes swollen and cannot be straightened (locked). This settles over a few weeks but subsequently repeat episodes of swelling, locking or giving-way may occur. Between attacks there may be little to see. If a cartilage tear is suspected arthroscopy is arranged. The surgeon inserts a fine, fibre-optic telescope into the knee under local anaesthetic, through which he can look around the whole joint. Many cartilage tears can be treated at the same time by cutting away the torn bit with tools passed down the telescope.

Bursitis

Bursae may become inflamed through repetitive wear, infection, or as part of an inflammatory arthritis such as rheumatoid, because joints and bursase have similar lining cells. The ones which give most trouble are:

1.   Pre-patellar bursitis (housemaid's knee), in front of and below the knee.
2.   Trochanteric bursitis, overlying the bony prominence of the upper outer part of the thigh, may mimic sciatica or hip disease.
3.   Psoas bursitis, felt in the groin, is even more similar to hip joint pain.
4.   Ischial bursitis, felt at the bony point deep in the buttock on which we sit.
5.   Achilles bursitis, felt behind the heel deep to the Achilles tendon.
6.   Olecranon bursitis (boozer's elbow). The olecranon bursa is visible as a sizeable swelling behind the elbow in some people and not uncommonly becomes inflamed. Lumps behind the elbow may form in gout or rheumatoid arthritis and distinguishing them from olecranon bursitis can be difficult.

Bursitis is usually treated by injecting the sac with steroid unless infection is present. The affected bursae are occasionally removed surgically.

Shoulder Joint Problems

Referred Pain

Pain around the shoulder is common and has many causes including arthritis, tendonitis and bursitis. It raises the problem that patients and doctors often mean different things when they use the same word. Patients usually think of their shoulder as the point of the shoulder and the region from there to the root of the neck across the shoulder blade. In fact, pain at these sites never arises in the shoulder joint but usually in the neck, whereas disease of the shoulder joint and tendons is felt in the muscle of the outer upper arm and may extend to the wrist. These are examples of referred pain, where pain arising in deep tissues such as joints cannot accurately be localised there but is felt in those muscles which share the same nerve supply, even though they may have moved some way apart during embryonic development.

Frozen Shoulder (Capsulitis)

In this common condition, the capsule of the shoulder becomes inflamed for no known reason and tightens up around the joint. Movement is severely restricted and initially it is very, very painful. In spite of the enthusiastic claims of some doctors, recovery from frozen shoulder is rarely shortened by treatment. Initially, in the most painful stage, rest and slings are sensible, but tablets rarely help. Some use steroid injections but I find these of little benefit in treating true frozen shoulder. Later, as the pain eases, physiotherapy may improve some patients, but even if nothing is done, the shoulder will always recover completely in eighteen months or less and the condition will never recur on the same side.

Rotator Cuff Tendonitis and Subacromial Bursitis

Here again pain is felt in the upper arm, but unlike in capsulitis the doctor can gently move the shoulder through a full range even if you find it too painful to move it actively yourself. The shoulder is a ball and socket joint and the three movements of rotating the arm outwards, inwards and away from the side are made by three muscles whose tendons converge on the shoulder to form an encircling, fibrous 'rotator cuff'. The tendons work through a narrow arch between the bones around the shoulder and may become abraded and sore. Pain is worst about half-way through the motion of lifting the arm as the tendon catches on the overlying bone, and may ease as the tendon has passed the narrow section and the arm is straightened up.

Treatment is by injecting steroid into the inflamed area but in young patients with recurrent trouble room can be made for the tendon by removing a small bit of the collar bone. In older patients the rotator cuff is very tatty and tends to rupture completely, but pain can again be relieved by injection. After about twelve months the patient learns to use other muscles to achieve a reasonable degree of function. The tissue of the cuff is too frail to be repaired at this age. Not surprisingly, there is a bursa between the rotator cuff and the overlying bone called the subacromial bursa. This may become inflamed, with symptoms very like rotator cuff tendonitis, and shows a good response to injection.

Miscellaneous Conditions

Dupuytren's Contracture

This is a gradual shortening of the fibrous tissue in the palm. A hard dimple is visible just below the base of the fourth and fifth fingers which in severe cases gradually become bent and tethered to the palm. Such patients can be treated surgically with variable success. Alcohol was once thought to be the cause, but this is not the case.

Garrod's Pads

These are fleshy pads over the knuckles which must be distinguished from gouty or rheumatoid nodules. They are harmless.

Musculo-skeletal Chest Pain

Sharp central chest pain often afflicts young people who naturally then worry about their hearts. A cardiogram or X-ray may be done to reassure, but lots of tests only worsen anxiety. The problem may be due to irritation of nerve roots in the thoracic spine or arises from the joints between rib and breastbone (costo-chondritis). It is rarely serious and usually gives no trouble once explained.

Fibrositis (Fibromyalgia)

Fibrositis was a term used to explain widespread muscular aches and tenderness. You may recall adverts for patent medicines with diagrams locating 'trigger points' which were thought to be foci of inflammation in the muscle. Even careful examination under the microscope fails to reveal inflammation at these sites and the term fibrositis is now frowned upon.

Most aches in muscles probably represent referred pain from the spine. Even so, many patients do complain of tender areas in muscle which are sometimes eased by massage or local injection, and for some the problem completely disrupts their lives. Since there is no imflammatory basis the term fibrositis has been changed to fibromyalgia (muscular aching). Many doctors remain sceptical but others feel it is a true disease which has its basis in altered pain sensation – pain amplification. Sleep pattern is disturbed and patients may be lethargic. Sympathy, explanation and reassurance can help a lot but sometimes low doses of anti-depressant drugs are used. This does not imply that the patient has a mental disorder. Anti-depressants probably relieve depressed patients by altering transmission of signals between nerve cells and in low dose they can do this in 'pain pathways' and 'sleep centres'.

Repetitive Strain Injury (RSI)

This is a fashionable term, better known in the USA and Australia than in Britain, referring to pain in the soft tissues, allegedly arising from repetitive strains at work. Some of the conditions already described can be related to occupational strains but they are identifiable conditions. The problem with RSI is that the diagnosis is being applied to complaints of pain in the absence of demonstrable tissue damage. In Australia where it is a major national issue, huge compensation costs are involved and expensive changes in work practices have been negotiated. Some have become chronically and disproportionately disabled by apparently minor conditions, a common feature when patients are 'over-investigated'. Naturally there is a suspicion that in some cases issues of compensation or malingering may prolong symptoms.

3
Osteo-arthritis

Osteo-arthritis (OA) is the commonest arthritis and a very old one, being found in fossils, Egyptian mummies and skeletons of men and animals. Five million people in Britain have symptoms of it and many more would show signs of osteo-arthritis if examined or X-rayed, but are unaware of it. People are frequently made very anxious by a comment that they have arthritis or that their joints are wearing out on the basis of an X-ray, imagining it the first sign of a crippling disorder which will spread to other joints, whereas actually many of them will never develop symptoms.

Osteo-arthritis has traditionally been thought of as a degenerative disease of ageing joints and is usually described pessimistically as 'wear and tear' arthritis. Certainly OA is increasingly common with age, but so are heart disease and cancer and we don't throw up our hands about them and say 'it's inevitable'. Changes in osteo-arthritic joints are not the same as those in ageing joints and many old people do not develop OA. There are racial differences too, and some types run in families. Normal vigorous exercise of a joint does not cause osteo-arthritis, although trauma which disrupts the joint surface may do. Similarly, damage to the joint surface by another disease such as rheumatoid arthritis may be such that even after that disease settles down, osteo-arthritic changes may progress to distort the joint further. Some people with rare inherited abnormalities of body chemistry are prone to OA, suggesting they may have intrinsic weaknesses in the composition of their joint tissues.

These facts have led to a new view of osteo-arthritis in which multiple causes, inherited and environmental, combine to produce the final changes in cartilage and bone which we call osteo-arthritis and which destroy the joint. In each sufferer some factors will be important and others may not be present. This approach holds the promise that with better understanding of these processes we may design drugs that interfere with some of them.

CHANGES IN THE OSTEO-ARTHRITIC JOINT

Before there is anything to see the composition of the joint cartilage changes, with decreases in normal proteoglycan molecules and increases in the content of water and destructive enzymes. The first visible change is flaking of the surface layer of cartilage over part of the joint so it becomes roughened. This may not progress, but if it does, deeper splits develop in the cartilage, usually over years, until underlying bone is exposed over part or all of the joint surface. Normal cartilage is not visible on X-ray so this stage of OA shows as narrowing of the gap between the bones of the joint. The bone at the margin of the joint may develop outgrowths called osteophytes, which may be frustrated attempts to remodel the joint. These can produce dramatic X-rays but have little relation to the severity of symptoms. With time, in severe cases, the touching raw bone surfaces wear away painfully and the joint becomes increasingly distorted and unstable. In osteo-arthritis the synovial lining is thickened and mildly inflamed and joint fluid accumulates to form an effusion which, in stretching the capsule and ligaments, contributes to this instability.

SYMPTOMS

Although inflammatory changes occur in osteo-arthritic joints these are usually mild and a distinction is correctly made between the essentially non-inflammatory nature of OA and the often intense inflammation of active rheumatoid. Osteo-arthritic patients may be a bit stiff in the morning or after sitting but soon shake it off and generally do not feel ill in themselves, whereas rheumatoid sufferers usually have prolonged stiffness and aching in the morning and feel unwell. Rheumatoid is a disease of the whole system and can make the sufferer tired and anaemic, sometimes damaging organs other than joints. Osteo-arthritic patients may feel depressed, crotchety and frustrated because of pain and loss of freedom but they are not ill.

Osteo-arthritis may begin at any time in adult life, usually as a niggling discomfort in a single joint with little to see. Most of us will experience this at some time. The pain is worse after use and at the end of the day. Most sufferers have three or four affected joints.

In spite of its reputation as a progressive wear and tear disease some joints never get much worse and any progress is usually slow, with even very painful joints settling down for long periods for no apparent reason. Of course, with time, in some patients one or more joints may become more severely damaged, unstable and painful.

There is also a condition called generalised osteo-arthritis (GOA) which mainly affects middle-aged women, some of whom have a family history of it in female relatives. These patients show small hard lumps on the joints at the end of the fingers called Heberden's nodes and similar swellings on the middle joints of the fingers called Bouchard nodes; these are just osteophytes. Some, but not all, patients with GOA have more widespread osteo-arthritis than the usual form. In the early stages of GOA inflammation in some joints may be more severe than is normally associated with OA and can cause much pain and visible redness at the joints. Fortunately this phase is brief, perhaps lasting a couple of years or so, and although the lumps on the fingers remain, they become painless and do not reduce function.

TREATMENT

Once the essentially benign nature of osteo-arthritis has been explained many patients cope perfectly well without treatment or by using pain-killers and modifying their life-style a little. Using a stick or losing weight may help.

Although you should remain active, it is pointless to push a joint until it gets very sore. Exercise little and often is best, so break up walks or shopping trips with a sit down to rest. If you do overdo it, you will not do any harm; the worst that will happen is that the joint will hurt more for a day or so.

I rarely use physiotherapy for osteo-arthritis except to retrain and build up disused muscles around a painful joint to improve stability, or perhaps prepare for joint replacement. The anti-inflammatory effect of steroid injections is also less effective in OA, although they can be surprisingly helpful early on. Once a joint has become badly damaged it is best to seek a surgical solution if possible and this should not be delayed until the last possible moment.

COMMON JOINT PROBLEMS

Not all joints are equally affected in osteo-arthritis. The shoulder, for example, is rarely involved.

Base of the Thumb

This joint forms the transition from the wrist into the smooth curve of the thumb and as osteo-arthritis develops it becomes square shaped, so that together with the Heberden's and Bouchard's nodes on the fingers it gives a characteristic appearance to the hands of people with GOA (*see* Fig 4). The joint may be quite troublesome in the early years but injections are helpful at this site and can last a long time. Thumb splints are also practical and beneficial. Surgical options are not very satisfactory and are rarely needed.

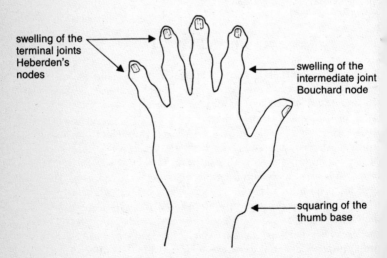

swelling of the terminal joints Heberden's nodes

swelling of the intermediate joint Bouchard node

squaring of the thumb base

Fig 4 A typical hand in generalised osteo-arthritis.

The Knee

The patello-femoral joint between kneecap and thigh bone is often involved in osteo-arthritis, even in young people, causing unnerving grating sounds and discomfort as the knee moves. It is rarely a serious problem and is best tolerated.

The main joint of the knee between femur and tibia may benefit from physiotherapy to build up the thigh muscles (quadriceps exercises). This will stabilise the joint and make walking less painful. In the early stages, steroid injections may give relief and like all osteo-arthritic joints it can settle for months or years without warning. Splints rarely provide adequate support for the knee. Swellings of the back of the joint capsule (Baker's cysts) can sometimes occur in OA (*see* Chapter 5 for a fuller description).

The idea of a knee joint replacement worries many patients who have the impression that it is a risk and does not work. This is not true. The immediate results are usually excellent and many of my patients are happy with knees put in over ten years ago. The point is that, unlike hip joints, knee replacements have not yet settled on the best design. The surgeon cannot therefore quote a long experience for any particular technique. The more recent knee replacements simply cap the damaged joint surfaces without the need for long fixing spikes into the thigh and shin bones, which tended to work loose.

The Hip

Patients think of the hip as the upper, outer thigh and buttock. Pain in that region rarely comes from the hip joint but nearly always from the spine, whereas true hip pain is felt deep in the groin and may be referred down the thigh to the knee or even felt entirely in the knee. Patients often argue bitterly with the surgeon who intends to replace their hip to relieve pain in their knee. The results of hip replacement are so good and patients are on their feet again so quickly that once pain is significantly disruptive a surgeon should be consulted. Obviously there is a place for delaying tactics in the very young, where they might be expected to outlive the life of the joint or in those where operation carries unacceptable medical risks. Old age is no barrier.

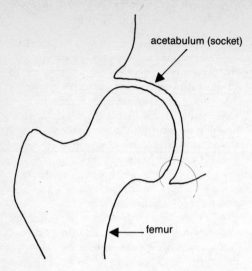

Fig 5   A normal hip joint (the capsule is not shown).

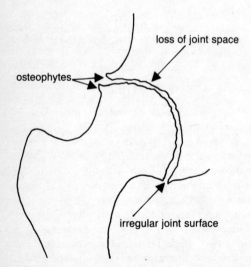

Fig 6   Changes in the osteo-arthritic hip joint.

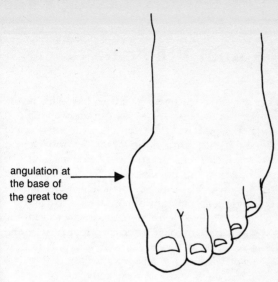

angulation at
the base of
the great toe

Fig 7   Hallux valgus.

The Big Toe (Hallux)

Osteo-arthritis of the big toe is incredibly common. The joint may
just stiffen and be unable to extend (hallux rigidus) or may bend
over towards the other toes, producing an angulation at the base of
the big toe which rubs against the shoes (hallux valgus) (*see* Fig 7).
A protective bursa develops at this site to form the common
bunion. The area may become reddened and mistaken for gout but
the pain is not sufficiently severe for gout and is more constant and
nagging. Care with footwear and padded insoles are often sufficient
as treatment but there is a range of good surgical solutions for those
who need them.

4
Spinal Problems

Back pain is a symptom, not a disease, and so like pain in the abdomen it can have many causes. There are some well-defined conditions affecting the spine but these only account for a small fraction of cases – and in the vast majority of attacks of back pain we do not know from which spinal structures the pain arises. Most rheumatologists admit this and use the term 'non-specific back pain' for this group. Now, this is not an attractive position for a specialist to adopt, and there are many other doctors, fringe practitioners and well-meaning friends of the patient who will fill the vacuum of knowledge with confident assertions about cause and treatment. I am not sure that all they say is nonsense, only that we have no proof for any of it. Contrary to popular belief, there is a lot of research going on into back pain and the group of conditions for which we have no answers should become smaller.

THE SPINAL STRUCTURE

The spine is a column of individual vertebral bones piled up like draughts. The basic structure of each vertebra is the same throughout the spine, but they are modified to cope with different functions at each level. For example, the vertebrae in the neck (cervical region) are small and light, and the joints between them allow movement in most directions, whereas the low back or lumbar region has more massive vertebrae which can cope with lifting tasks but allow only limited movement other than flexion. The shape of a typical vertebra is shown in Fig 8. There is a solid block of bone in front (the body) to which is fused an arch of bone behind. The series of arches forms the spinal canal down which the spinal cord runs, surrounded by a protective fluid-filled sack of membranes (meninges). Between each adjacent pair of vertebrae a pair of spinal nerve roots joins the spinal cord, one at each side. These roots contain a two-way traffic of sensory fibres entering the brain

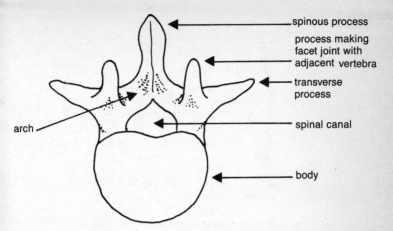

Fig 8   A typical vertebra.

and motor fibres leaving the brain to work the muscles.

Fig 9 illustrates a short segment of the spinal column to show how the vertebrae are joined together. Between the bodies is an inter-vertebral disc. The core of this disc is a jelly-like substance con-tained by a thick capsule of collagen fibres intermeshed like the husk of a coconut to provide an excellent shock absorber between the bones.

The vertebrae are also joined by stout projections of bone which make synovial joints with each other – the facet joints. Variations in the shape and angle of these facet joints dictate the type of move-ment possible in the different spinal regions. The whole interlinked column is further bound together by long and short ligaments and by the massive anti-gravity muscles of the back which act like guy ropes to resist our natural tendency to tip forward.

Although the normal spine is straight viewed from the front, there are natural curves from front to back so that the lumbar region curves forwards (lumbar lordosis) and so does the cervical spine. The intervening thoracic (or dorsal) spine has a compen-satory backwards curve. Temporary alterations of the normal cur-vature may result from muscle spasm during attacks of pain. Below the lumbar spine the vertebrae rapidly shrink in size and are fused

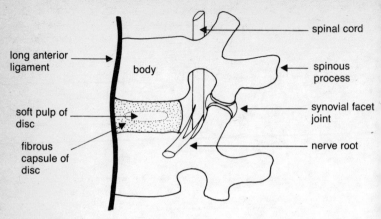

long anterior ligament

body

spinal cord

spinous process

soft pulp of disc

synovial facet joint

fibrous capsule of disc

nerve root

Fig 9   Two adjacent vertebral bodies.

to form the sacrum which is joined on each side, through the sacro-iliac joint, to the ring of pelvic bones (*see* Fig 13).

NON-SPECIFIC BACK PAIN

This condition makes up over 90 per cent of all back pain. Most attacks come on fairly rapidly and are relatively short-lived, lasting just a few days or weeks. They virtually all clear up even if not treated. An attack may arise 'out of the blue' or may follow lifting or twisting, or a heavy day in the garden. Pain is felt widely across the low back rather than over the spine and may extend into buttock and thigh. This is lumbago, i.e. pain in the lumbar region. The low back loses its natural curve and stiffens. The patient tends to walk bent and resents further bending or straightening, 'my back locked' being the usual complaint. Rest in a comfortable position helps, but may not be easy to achieve. Changing position hurts but as the sufferer hobbles about he usually loosens up, only to stiffen again after being stationary.

Causes

Some of the more dramatic attacks of lumbago very much resemble the features of a ruptured disc but without sciatica. Careful questioning of the patient may bring out intermittent symptoms of sciatic type pain, or tingling, and I imagine such patients have indeed suffered a minor disc prolapse. However, most acute cases of back pain are not due to a 'slipped' disc which 'goes back' or is 'pushed back' by manipulation. Discs do not slip, they rupture. The jelly-like pulp bursts through a rent in the capsule like putting your thumb on a soft chocolate. The only way you could put it back would be to run the film backwards. Ruptured discs heal slowly by scar formation and shrinkage.

There is no doubt that some patients with acute pain get dramatic, sudden relief as they are being manipulated. This is often interpreted as freeing a facet joint that has got stuck but we cannot know this for certain. No one ends up on the post-mortem slab from acute back pain so we cannot look and see, and each pair of vertebrae are joined by several interdependent facet joints so that one joint cannot be moved in isolation. Sometimes injections to numb the facet joints can help.

Patients are frequently told that they have 'arthritis' of the spine on the basis of X-rays. This is often rubbish and is extremely worrying for the patient because they believe the problem will spread and cripple them. X-ray changes in the spine (spondylosis) begin to appear in most of us by early middle age and become increasingly likely as we grow older, so that any pain-free person of the same age is as likely to have an abnormal spinal X-ray as the patient. Studies have shown that the severity of back pain bears no relation to the amount of X-ray changes and the frequency of back pain is highest in middle age, then becomes less, while the X-ray continues to worsen with age. Another reason I dislike the term 'arthritis of the spine' is that the diagnosis is usually based on the presence of osteophytes (*see* Chapter 3). These arise from the body of the vertebrae, where there are no moving joints, and merely reflect bone remodelling. Of course, the synovial facet joints can become osteo-arthritic, and this presumably explains why injections into them help some people, but most true arthritic conditions such as rheumatoid do not cause low back problems.

The remaining possibility is that acute non-specific back pain is due to strains of ligaments and muscles and since we all have experience of such injuries in the limbs, it seems likely that they may account for similar problems in the back. This is a common-sense argument but none the worse for that. Muscle spasm is a common feature of back ache, where it may be a secondary effect to splint the tender spine.

So, acute attacks of back pain tend to be brief and self-limiting, and although they may recur and vary in severity they do not inevitably get worse as time goes by and patients never become 'crippled'. Most people suffer less trouble as they approach retirement age.

A smaller number of patients suffer chronic, non-specific back pain, either as low-grade discomfort punctuated by acute attacks of pain, or as more constant, nagging pain. This condition tends to be affected by the same factors that influence acute back pain. The majority are perfectly capable of coping with this problem once its benign nature is explained, but for a small percentage of chronic back pain sufferers their world seems to come to an end and unemployment and depression ensue. Their apparently disproportionate reaction to an essentially non-serious condition is variously interpreted as 'having a low pain threshold', 'pain amplification syndrome' (*see* Chapter 2), depression or neurosis. I do not know which is correct, but the fact remains that for such patients the outlook is bleak. Multi-disciplinary teams of doctors, pain experts, fringe therapists and psychiatrists are being set up to help, but most of these patients trudge endlessly from clinic to clinic seeking cause and treatment.

Although this extreme reaction is unusual, many people are unduly concerned by back pain, and a few further points may help to reassure:

1. Pain from the lumbar spine is not usually felt over the vertebrae but in the loin, buttock or thighs as far as the knees. Patients interpret this as kidney pain or hip disease and cannot believe it can be due to local causes in the back.
2. There is confusion between spine and spinal cord, and fear that the back may snap or the patient become paralysed. The spine is no such fragile thing and the usual forms of back pain carry no

risk of paralysis, whatever you do in the way of work or exercise –
it will simply hurt.

3.   Some are worried they may have a tumour. Such sinister
causes are very rare, nearly always raising suspicion at once, and
they can usually be confirmed or denied very easily.

4.   The lack of certainty about the cause of most back pain and the
failure of treatment to improve on natural healing leads to patients
receiving conflicting advice and being offered a wide range of
empirical treatments. This leads them to question why no one can
find out what is going on and why things are not getting better.
Could the doctor have missed something serious? I hope this
chapter has helped calm some such worries.

Treatment

If you are not sure what causes a condition, treatment has to be
shrewd guesswork, modified by past experience. A recent large-
scale study shows that the traditional treatment of a few days bed-
rest is as effective as any other. Take up whatever position you find
comfortable and use a bed with a firm base but a comfortable mat-
tress. Most so-called orthopaedic beds are too hard, too expensive,
and have never been near an orthopaedic surgeon.

There are many other treatments on offer, including corsetry,
exercises, manipulations, traction, heat pads, acupuncture and a
variety of electrical devices. Those that have been evaluated in controlled trials of large numbers of patients show them to be little better than doing nothing, and many treatments have never been
tested at all. No treatment has been shown to prevent recurrence of
back pain. Losing weight, swimming and any other exercise have
no preventive value other than providing the benefits of involving
the patient in self-care and improving general health.

Of course, these treatments do appear to help *some* patients or
they would not continue in use. The trouble with evidence from
personal experience in particular patients, so-called anecdotal
evidence, is that it takes no account of the natural tendency of the
illness to clear up on its own. Treatments and practitioners
therefore acquire unjustified reputations if they happen to be
treating the patient at the time when he would have been recover-
ing anyway. The other explanation is that the patients who respond

to a particular treatment have a particular sort of back pain which we cannot yet distinguish. Again, only careful trials with large numbers of patients, which carefully record the details of each, can ever hope to show this and allow better selection of treatment.

Non-specific Back Pain and Work

I am often asked for advice about work by patients and employers, but this is a very problematic area. A recent article listed nearly a hundred predisposing factors involving work, quoted by five leading authorities on back pain. Nearly two-thirds of these had no supporting evidence or were based on a single study. Only thirteen of the factors were agreed by the majority of the experts. These were:

1. Age.
2. Muscle strength relative to the task.
3. Physical fitness.
4. Previous back pain.
5. Work experience of the task.
6. Psycho-social factors.
7. Heavy physical work.
8. Prolonged sitting.
9. Heavy handling work.
10. Loading or frequent lifting.
11. Rotation of the trunk.
12. Pushing or pulling.
13. Vibration.

Statistics on occupational back pain are usually collected for company purposes, such as sick pay. They do not measure the frequency of back pain but the frequency with which people stop work because of it. This is likely to be influenced by prevailing conditions of job security, unemployment, social security provision, the policy of the company or union on injury reporting, and criteria of fitness for the job. Although manual workers and nurses have high rates of work lost through back pain, this may not mean that they suffer more back trouble, but simply that such workers cannot carry on their physically demanding work when they get backache, whereas in a lighter job they might have continued to work on with the same problem. High rates of work lost through backache also afflict sedentary office workers but perhaps such occupations attract the less physically robust. On the other hand, research has shown that the stresses on the discs can be considerably reduced by seating offering good support, so in principle well-designed furniture and equipment might reduce the incidence of backache.

Faced with such uncertainty it is hard to give authoritative advice. If you suffer frequent backache you are unlikely to be able to continue for long in heavy work and, if possible, a change of job would be wise. It is also common sense to look at your home and work life and to change techniques or equipment if a particular activity regularly upsets your back. Keep generally fit and if you get an attack of severe back pain, rest for a few days if possible. If you know a treatment that helps you, such as a corset or hanging off the banister, use it.

RUPTURED (PROLAPSED) INTERVERTEBRAL DISC

This is typically a condition of young adults and the middle-aged, although it can occur in the elderly, where it tends to show a different pattern. The onset usually follows lifting or twisting injudiciously. Initially, the back pain may be only moderate but within hours or days there is severe lumbago. The pain extends into the leg, typically the whole length, from the buttock down the back of the thigh and calf to the foot, and there may be sensations of numbness or pins and needles, suggesting a nerve is being irritated. This is sciatica (pain in the distribution of the sciatic nerve) and it is virtually always due to a ruptured disc pressing on the adjacent nerve root. We know this because some patients go to surgery where we get visible proof. The pain is often made worse when the patient coughs or sneezes, since this raises the pressure around the nerve roots. Bending and changing position may be agonising. By examining the reflexes, muscles and sensation, it may be possible to detect the exact nerve root being irritated. Although most patients will have an X-ray and a blood test, these are nearly always unhelpful – their main purpose is to reassure.

Attacks of sciatica usually clear up within three months and nearly all sufferers will be back to normal in a year. Many patients are happy to sit things out once reassurances and explanations are given. Corsets, simple pain-killers and muscle relaxants, and bed rest all seem to help some people, but I do not prescribe physiotherapy if there are signs of nerve pressure. A common modern treatment is the epidural injection (EDI), often performed on an outpatient and taking only a few minutes. Under local anaesthetic a small volume of steroid solution in salty water is injected to shrink the inflammation around the damaged disc and so free the nerve. I have never seen any side-effects from this, other than, occasionally, a day or so of worse discomfort. It is very effective in relieving many episodes of sciatic pain but does not usually help large disc prolapses. It does nothing for simple back pain either. No one can predict if and when a repeat attack of sciatica may occur but many patients have only one attack.

If the attack is very severe or prolonged, or if attacks recur frequently, surgery is considered. This is preceded by a special X-ray, a radiculogram, in which an X-ray dye is put into the fluid around the spinal cord and nerves by an extension of the EDI technique. Several pictures are taken in different positions, with the patient tilted on a table, so the process takes a little while. Sometimes the patient will stay in hospital for one night feeling a little sick or with a headache. The X-ray shows whether part of the disc has pressed on to a nerve root. If so, it can be removed, usually through a small incision and without removing a lot of bone, as used to be the case.

Results of this operation for sciatica are excellent, with rapid relief of pain and only a short stay in hospital. Operations on the back have gained a bad reputation because they used to be done in large numbers purely for back pain, on the wrong assumption that this was usually due to disc trouble. The results were therefore very disappointing. Patients are often puzzled and frustrated when their doctors refuse to consider surgery for even severe, chronic back pain, while they know a friend who is absolutely delighted with an operation on his back. The point is that the friend will have had sciatica as his main problem, not backache. Very occasionally some surgeons may consider fusing two adjacent vertebrae together across a damaged disc when they think this is the cause of back pain. Others are not so keen and there is a risk that stiffening part of the spine will stress the nearby normal discs. Another technique for a single disc problem is to inject a chemical into it, under local anaesthetic, to dissolve the disc (discolysis).

Disc Disease in the Elderly

It is rare to get a first attack of sciatica in old age, when it is usually the discs in the upper lumbar spine which rupture. This is probably because the lower ones which cause sciatica have already worn away. The higher lumbar nerve roots run in front of the thigh across the hip joint, so pain and tingling are felt in this area. This is called cruralgia (the Latin *crura* means groins). Many non-specialists are unaware of this condition and misdiagnose osteo-arthritis of the hip. The condition does very well with time or EDI and rarely needs surgery.

PAIN IN THE NECK

Pain in the neck is only a little less common than low back pain but I will discuss it briefly since most of the general comments about low back pain also apply to the cervical spine.

Acute disc rupture is not as common in the neck as in the low back and most attacks of pain are in the non-specific category. Again, you should not be misled by changes on the X-ray (cervical spondylosis) into assuming that the pain is due to arthritis. Pain arising in the cervical spine is felt across the muscles of the upper back and shoulder and into the arms, so many patients believe they have shoulder trouble or 'fibrositis'. The pain often extends up the back of the head or may be referred to the forehead. Naturally, a number of people consult their doctor with great anxiety that they have high blood pressure or a brain tumour. In cases of disc prolapse, when a nerve root is irritated, neuralgic symptoms are felt in the arm or hand analogous to the situation in sciatica.

Some older patients experience giddy spells, especially on turning the head. This is said to be due to brief kinking of the blood vessels to the brain as they run through small bony canals in the cervical vertebrae which have been distorted by 'wear and tear' in the neck. I am not sure this is the exact cause, although the attacks

39

certainly suggest that brain blood flow is temporarily disturbed. This sounds pretty awful but the symptom is actually not very serious.

Most attacks of neckache come on suddenly, producing a stiff neck with restricted movement, and clear up within two weeks. True disc rupture is usually much more painful and may be severe for six weeks before gradually resolving. Fortunately cervical disc rupture rarely recurs, but non-specific neck pain usually does. As with low back pain some suffer chronic discomfort and while most cope, a minority become obsessed.

Acute neck pain may be treated with rest in a collar or by shaping the pillows to give support. Muscle relaxants may give a night's rest but I find anti-inflammatory drugs useless. There is also evidence that early mobilisation or manual traction is good for many acutely painful necks but it should not be used if nerve roots are involved. Surgeons are very reluctant to tackle the cervical spine, even when nerve entrapment is obvious.

Rheumatoid arthritis attacks the neck quite commonly, unlike the rest of the spine, but sufferers have other features of the illness, so it is not likely to be the cause of a pain in the neck in otherwise well patients.

PAIN IN THE THORACIC SPINE

This is much less common than pain elsewhere but its features are similar. A particular worry for some of these patients is the perception of pain in front of the chest, suggesting heart disease.

SPECIFIC SPINAL PROBLEMS
Scheurmann's Disease

Scheurmann's disease is a condition of the thoracic spine in teenagers where part of the developing cartilages crumble and a kyphosis develops. Everyone becomes very concerned, but the back straightens again and only a few suffer discomfort from time to time in later life.

Spondylolysis and Spondylolisthesis

A spondylolysis is a defect in the bony arch of a vertebra and is often congenital. Some occurrences follow trauma, possibly because there may also be an inherited local weakness of the arch. The defect may allow one vertebra to slip forward on another. This is called spondylolisthesis which can also be due to severe osteo-arthritis of the facet joints. A slip in the spine sounds horrendous but it is usually slight and even major slips seen on X-ray may cause no problems for the patient, or can be helped by a corset. Since the abnormalities are common, their presence on the X-ray does not necessarily mean that they are the cause of your pain, so a decision to stabilise the slip by surgery can require fine judgement.

Spinal Stenosis and Spinal Claudication

Spondylolisthesis is one cause of a narrowing of the lower part of the spinal canal (spinal stenosis). This may put pressure on nerve roots within the canal and often the symptoms of buttock or back pain, or sciatica, come on only after exercise. This is called spinal claudication (the Latin *claudio* means I limp). Claudication is much more usually due to hardening of the arteries to the legs and some patients have this as well, so sorting the problem out can be difficult. If established, spinal claudication is treated surgically.

Coccydinia

This is a condition of pain and tenderness at the lowermost tip of the spine in the cleft of the buttocks. It represents a fracture or dislocation of the tiny lowest vertebra, the coccyx. The pain can be quite miserable and usually is only partially relieved by cushions and local steroid injections, but it clears up within two years.

Osteoporotic Collapse

Osteoporosis is thinning of bone which is a feature of ageing especially prevalent in white women. A thin vertebra may suddenly collapse (a crush fracture) for no reason, or after even a slight shock such as a cough. The pain is sudden and severe and is made worse by coughing or sneezing, but eases gradually so that by about six weeks patients are pretty comfortable; they are usually out of pain by twelve weeks. In the painful stage, all you can do is rest, take pain-killing tablets or wear a corset. But once the pain allows, you should 'get moving' because the best way of slowing osteoporosis is by keeping active. Osteoporotic collapse higher up in the thoracic spine causes the 'Dowager's hump' of some elderly ladies.

Preventive treatment for osteoporosis is controversial. You should keep active and many advise calcium supplements, but not Vitamin D. Hormone replacement for a few years after the menopause will slow the rapid loss of bone at that time and will reduce the incidence of fractures. It seems to carry fewer risks than was previously believed.

Arachnoiditis

This is scarring around the spinal nerve roots. It can follow meningitis or back surgery, especially after repeat operations. It causes chronic discomfort and unfortunately there is as yet no effective treatment.

5

Rheumatoid Arthritis

Some rheumatologists prefer to call this condition rheumatoid disease since it is an inflammatory illness which can damage other organs as well. When the disease is active the patient suffers the non-specific effects of inflammation: tiredness, malaise, weight loss and anaemia. Although the progress of rheumatoid is very variable, in many people it goes on for a long time which makes it what doctors call a chronic disease (the Greek *chronos* means time). The frequency of rheumatoid arthritis in the population has probably been overestimated but may run at 1–2 per cent.

CAUSES

Perhaps the most frequent question I am asked by patients about rheumatoid or other arthritic conditions is 'what causes it?' It seems to be a basic human assumption that everything has a simple beginning at a point in time, yet whenever we enquire into causes of major disasters, for example, we find instead several factors which on their own are insufficient as causes but when coinciding produce far-reaching consequences. Curiously we never like such explanations and prefer simple concepts of disease and its causes, such as 'the weather', 'diet' or 'stress'. But no illness is like that: most adults have antibodies in their blood to german measles or mumps, but many were never aware of being ill. A fall in an elderly lady with osteoporosis might break her hip, whereas I might only be bruised. The development of a disease always involves many factors, as we have already seen in osteo-arthritis, and rheumatoid is no exception.

The present view of the cause of rheumatoid arthritis is that a foreign organism, probably a virus, infects an individual who is constitutionally incapable of dealing with it in the normal way. The usual inflammatory response to the organism is prolonged and perverted, perhaps because host tissues are altered in the course of

43

the infection and are no longer recognised as self, so that a chronic, inappropriate, auto-immune inflammatory process is set up. This is not an immediately obvious conclusion, so what is the evidence for it?

There is certainly major immunological disturbance in rheumatoid disease. The inflamed synovium of rheumatoid joints contain large numbers of immunologically active cells and many of the drugs which are most effective in controlling the disease are toxic to these cells, suppressing immune activity. About three-quarters of rheumatoid patients have in their blood auto-antibodies which bind to their own antibody proteins. These auto-antibodies are called rheumatoid factors and patients who possess them are called sero-positive. The fluctuating level of rheumatoid factors in the blood of any one patient bears no relation to disease activity; rheumatoid factors are also found in other diseases and become increasingly prevalent in healthy people as they age, so most rheumatologists feel they simply tell us that something immunological is going on, rather than causing the disease.

Rheumatoid patients often fail to show an inflammatory reaction if the skin is injected with foreign proteins. The normal skin reaction is an example of cell-mediated immunity, a function of T cells. The production of antibodies such as rheumatoid factors is a function of B cells, whose activity can be suppressed by other types of T cells. We know that the ratio of helper T cells to suppressor T cells is abnormal in rheumatoid, so a picture emerges of defective T cell activity as being central in the pathology, although this will certainly prove to be too simple.

We know then that the immunological system is haywire in rheumatoid, but no one has yet found an organism to act as the trigger, so this part of the idea remains a guess. It is a good guess, though, because similar mechanisms are now known in some other diseases. This does not mean you can catch rheumatoid from sufferers – they are not infectious.

There is a higher frequency of the HLA DR4 gene in patients with rheumatoid compared with the normal population and HLA DR genes are especially important in the cell to cell interactions which generate the immune response. This is good evidence that individual susceptibility is important. The expression of rheumatoid in an individual is also influenced by their sex and hormonal status – it is more common in women and becomes quiet during pregnancy, recurring after birth of the child.

Obviously we are nowhere near the whole story and with further knowledge other favoured contenders for a causative role, such as diet, climate, stress, etc. will probably all be shown to play a part. However, I am sure it will be only a part. There is now ample evidence to make the simplistic idea of a single 'cause', so beloved of the fringe practitioner, most improbable.

CHANGES IN THE RHEUMATOID JOINT

Unlike the mild inflammatory changes in osteo-arthritic joints, the synovial lining in active rheumatoid arthritis is extremely inflamed and thickened. Aggregates of immunologically active plasma cells and lymphocytes can be seen, which co-operate to produce the rheumatoid factors as well as mediator molecules which attract large numbers of polymorph 'pus' cells, with their destructive enzymes, and huge effusions of synovial fluid develop, rich in polymorphs. Macrophages are also heavily represented in the rheumatoid synovium and contribute their own tissue-destroying enzymes. The inflamed synovium encroaches on the smooth cartilage surface of the joint and gradually destroys it and the underlying bone. Not all patients develop bone destruction of this sort, but in those that do the nibbling away of the bone may be seen on X-ray as 'erosions'.

A joint severely affected by the rheumatoid process will be swollen, tender, warm and even reddened. It will inevitably lose function so it shows a 'full house' of classical inflammatory features, reflecting the immunological turmoil beneath. A fine needle inserted into such a joint will release freely flowing fluid, cloudy with polymorph cells – an inflammatory effusion – quite unlike the sticky, clear fluid of osteo-arthritis. All these features tell the doctor that the patient has active synovitis. Not surprisingly, in a joint badly disrupted by such inflammation osteo-arthritic changes may continue to damage the joint even after the rheumatoid activity declines.

This description is pretty horrid so it is important to keep a sense of proportion. Not all the joints will be affected, and not all those that are will have the extreme activity described here. Even those that do can be settled down in most patients.

GENERAL SYMPTOMS

Rheumatoid arthritis is unpredictable in the way it starts, the way it progresses and in its response to treatment in any individual patient. Attempts to describe the illness are therefore unnecessarily worrying for those destined to have only mild or moderate disease. Bear this in mind as I start by outlining the scope of the illness and later deal with problems in particular joints and other complications.

Rheumatoid arthritis may begin in childhood or very old age, but usually starts in early middle age. Women are affected more often than men but men are rather more at risk of the non-arthritic complications of the disease. It usually begins gradually but can explode into activity over a few days. Elderly patients often have a rapid onset, with more muscle aching than joint pain in a picture indistinguishable from polymyalgia rheumatica (*see* Chaper 6).

Rarely, the disease may start with involvement of organs other than the joints, fluid on the lung, for example, perhaps with severe general upset, weight loss and fever. More sinister diseases are often suspected until joint troubles begin or tests reveal the truth.

A palindrome is a puzzle – palindromic rheumatism is the name given to a form of arthritis which begins quite atypically with pain and swelling of one or two joints for perhaps only a few hours or days at a time before returning completely to normal. In about half of these patients a more persistent, typical rheumatoid picture will emerge, sometimes after many years.

Usually the earliest joints to give trouble are the knuckles and adjacent finger joints and the corresponding joints at the base of the toes which lie under the ball of the foot causing pain like walking on marbles. Synovitis may not be detectable in the joints at first, but in this early stage inflammation of the flexor tendon sheaths may be obvious. The patient's fingers swell like a bunch of bananas and cannot close to a fist. Involvement of shoulders, elbows, wrists, knees and ankles and, less often, hips may follow. A striking feature of rheumatoid is the symmetrical distribution of affected joints on

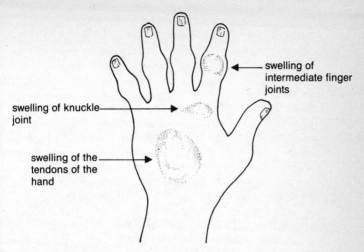

swelling of
intermediate finger
joints

swelling of knuckle
joint

swelling of the
tendons of the
hand

Fig 10   Early changes in rheumatoid arthritis.

each side of the body, although any pattern of joints can be affected and the illness may involve a single joint for years.

The active illness makes the patient feel unwell, occasionally out of proportion to the degree of joint involvement. They are tired, feel like they have flu, and are especially bad in the morning with aching stiffness (morning stiffness). Not so well recognised is a similar decline in the evening (vesperal stiffness).

The progress of the disease is just as variable and cannot be predicted with certainty at the start. About one quarter of patients will have a mild illness, sometimes very brief, while about two-thirds will have a more lasting illness, fluctuating in intensity, with periods of relatively normal health interrupted by flares in which pain, stiffness and fatigue get worse. Most of these patients will remain in employment and live full lives. An unfortunate 5 per cent will have serious, occasionally relentless, disease with severe joint damage and functional disability. When you attend the clinic these patients form an unrepresentative number of the patients you will see around you, because those who have mild or moderate illness will visit infrequently or not at all. By the law of averages you are far more likely to turn out to be one of the fortunate ones.

In most cases the active inflammatory phase of the illness burns out eventually. General ill health and morning stiffness lessen and anaemia corrects itself. Unfortunately, those joints which have been significantly damaged by the disease may continue to give pain and disability because of superimposed osteo-arthritic changes and instability.

For most patients the functional disability is as distressing as the pain, or more so. Loss of personal freedom plus the discomfort, frustrates and grinds down the personality and depression is common. This in turn lowers pain tolerance and motivation and a lapse into invalidism can occur, which antagonises friends and partners and strains relationships. So-called 'conventional' sexual activity is often given up as impossible or too painful. The onset of the disease in the peak earning years may lead to loss of income or unemployment and the financial burden can weigh heavily. The patient worries about the future and may meanwhile suffer disappointments as initial attempts at treatment take time to work, or fail, or cannot be tolerated because of side-effects.

MANAGEMENT OF RHEUMATOID ARTHRITIS

Rheumatoid arthritis is a classic example of a disease managed by a multi-disciplinary team approach. The most important member of the team is the patient because his personal resources of resilience, humour and intelligence are the most effective way of defeating this illness. Usually the rheumatologist becomes the co-ordinator, using his own skills and calling on those of colleagues in other medical specialities – surgeons, physiotherapists, occupational therapists, social workers, chiropodists, surgical fitters, layworkers and priests, as the need arises.

Decisions about management rarely have a right and wrong answer and often we can make a decision to do nothing but wait and see. 'When in doubt, do nowt' is a good motto in medicine. Often the right choice appears only in retrospect, after trial and error. All treatments carry side-effects which in most cases cannot be predicted for an individual patient; some drugs do not work for some people. I like patients to be aware of this uncertainty and to be involved in making the choices because I think that is the only way to maintain confidence when things are not going smoothly.

Management decisions at every stage begin with assessment of the patient and his disease.

Assessing Disease Activity

Assessing the severity of disease activity, strangely enough, is a most difficult matter. It is not the same as pain which may be severe in 'burnt out' disease because of mechanical factors, and it is not a matter of how ill the patient feels since this may be profoundly influenced by depression. Active inflammatory disease is suggested by prolonged morning stiffness, easy fatigue and by the presence of synovitis or by signs of new features developing such as new nodules or vasculitis.

We can be helped in this judgement by tests. The severity of anaemia tends to reflect disease activity, but we must be aware of other causes. A common test you will hear about is the ESR (erythrocyte sedimentation rate). This is influenced by the many substances which are released into the blood as mediators during active inflammation. Higher rates tend to indicate activity but it is a totally non-specific test and can be unreliable. The rate goes up during most illnesses and with age, and may be very high in some perfectly well people, so do not be obsessed with changes in your own ESR. The rheumatoid factor mentioned earlier is not useful for measuring activity, but it tends to predict more aggressive disease, so the doctor may be influenced by it to move on to more powerful treatment earlier than he otherwise might.

Obviously you will have X-rays taken, probably many times over in the early years to see if erosions are developing, increasing, or healing. Surprisingly, these too are not an absolutely reliable indicator of activity. Some people are erosion-free with florid synovitis, while patients with badly damaged joints may feel well and retain good function.

Armed with these various clues the doctor attempts to decide the degree of activity. Sometimes it is obvious, but often the clues conflict and judgement is very difficult.

Selecting Drug Treatment

Most patients will have some pain and the first line in treatment will be an anti-inflammatory medicine with aspirin-like actions which is designed to reduce stiffness, ease movement and, in lessening inflammation, reduce pain. A good proportion of the dose will be taken at bedtime to reduce the early morning increases in pain and stiffness, but patients on night work or with a different time pattern of pain should experiment with the timing of their tablets. Most patients also take simple pain-killers as well, such as paracetamol, since these do not interact with the anti-inflammatory medicines. Those with inactive or burnt-out disease often derive much of their pain from mechanical factors which may respond better to simple pain-killers than to anti-inflammatories, and there will be some who cannot safely use anti-inflammatories because of other conditions, stomach ulcers, for example.

If on this simple treatment the patient feels well, disease activity is slight, function is maintained and tests and X-rays are satisfactory, no further drug treatment will be offered. If, however, control is inadequate, and the disease active, the rheumatologist will consider adding 'second line' therapy. There are several of these agents such as chloroquine, gold, penicillamine and they are discussed, along with other rheumatic drugs, in Chapter 10. It is important to realise that these agents work in quite a different way to the anti-inflammatory drugs. They are slow, often taking several months to exert benefit, and during this time patients rightly become impatient. However, when they work they exert a much more profound dampening effect on the disease and in a good number of patients relieve active inflammation almost completely, improving blood tests and correcting the anaemia. For this reason they are also called 'disease modifying' drugs, implying that they actually tackle the fundamental processes of rheumatoid disease. Since we do not know what these processes are, nor how the drugs work, this claim is doubtful. It may be that they are just exceptionally powerful anti-inflammatory agents.

Any particular second line drug seems to work for only about two-thirds of patients and they have rather more frequent and serious side-effects than the simpler drugs, so some patients have to try several before one is tolerated and control is gained. This is obviously even more frustrating. It is because of the possible side-effects and the need to check the patient regularly with blood and urine tests that we do not use these powerful drugs on everyone with rheumatoid, and the decision to use them will be an individual one for each patient and each doctor. But if they are suggested, *do not* be put off by the risks.

Steroid therapy was widely used in rheumatoid about twenty to thirty years ago when the drugs first became available and there is no doubt that, given a big enough dose, a rapid and impressive improvement is achieved. With experience it was found that the doses necessary to maintain this well-being were such that the benefits were bought at too high a price in longer term side-effects. These began to outweigh the good as early as two years after starting treatment. Of course, even with steroids there are situations where the risks are smaller than the benefits, particularly for some serious complications of rheumatoid or when rapid relief is needed in a patient whose life and work is totally disrupted. Even in these situations we try to use the lowest effective dose for as short a time as possible, since we recognise that some patients can never bear to come off steroids once they have tasted the relief they bring in high doses.

Although patients with rheumatoid are usually managed as out-patients, there are times when the doctor will suggest hospital admission, especially when disease is active or at the onset of the illness. This is to combine the important benefit of complete bed-rest under nursing care with an opportunity to splint and inject joints, make management decisions, consult colleagues, try different drugs, and provide physiotherapy more quickly and efficiently than over a series of outpatient visits.

Assessing Individual Joints

Particular joints with especially severe pain or disability may benefit from individual attention in addition to the general treatment already outlined. Really tender joints are helped by resting them in splints and splinting may gradually reduce deformity in a joint such as a bent knee. Active synovitis can often be settled for months, by drawing off synovial fluid and injecting steroids into the joint. Steroid injections into joints do not have general side-effects on the body, but they can give a brief 'buzz' of well-being that is useful in dampening down a flare, or before a special social function. Radio-chemicals have been used for this and sometimes the joint lining is removed surgically. Burnt-out joints rarely benefit more than briefly from injections, but opportunities for well-tried surgical procedures should not be missed. Some joints will function less well than they ought because of wasting of the muscles that work them, through disuse. This is where the physiotherapist is invaluable, building up strength and confidence, perhaps in a hydrotherapy pool.

Assessing and Treating Complications

Rheumatoid disease and its complications, such as vasculitis, can affect several organs other than joints and it is important to look out for this and to distinguish these effects of the disease from the varied side-effects of the drugs used. Consequently, some patients will require the opinions of other specialists and investigations of heart, lungs, kidney or bone marrow from time to time.

Functional and Environmental Assessment

Ideally every visit to clinic should be used to get an update on how the patient is coping with everyday living: cooking, eating, bathing, toilet, etc., not forgetting work, social and sexual life. Obviously much disability in these areas may be helped by the success of treatments already described, but it is important to gauge mood and help depression if needed. This does not always mean drugs. Information may relieve ill-founded worries, letters and phone calls can untie bureaucratic irritations in financial, housing or employment matters. Finally, if you cannot change the patient – change their world, with modifications to footwear, clothing, home or car. Occupational therapists and social workers are the experts here.

RHEUMATOID IN PARTICULAR JOINTS

The Hand

Most rheumatoid patients will have hand involvement and any joint may be affected. In the early stages, inflammation of the flexor tendons is often more obvious and the patient cannot close the fist. Later triggering may develop (*see* Chapter 2). The extensor tendons may slip off to the side of the knuckle joints so that they pull on the fingers at an angle and contribute to the sideways deviation of the rheumatoid hand. Very inflamed tendons are weakened and liable to rupture, most often the extensor tendons of the fourth and fifth fingers as they run across the back of the rough, arthritic wrist. This causes inability to extend the fingers and usually requires urgent surgical repair.

Carpal tunnel compression of the median nerve (*see* Chapter 2) is particularly common in rheumatoid. This should be considered in all complaints of pain or disability in the hand as it is so easily treated.

The combination of arthritic damage and broken, misplaced, or lax tendons produces a variety of deformities in the joints. With few exceptions, rheumatoid patients tolerate these changes cheerfully because in spite of even advanced deformity, function can remain surprisingly good. Because of this, doctors are cautious about surgical attempts to replace hand joints or transplant tendons,

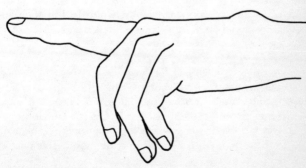

Fig 11   Ruptured extensor tendons in rheumatoid arthritis.

since often the functional result is no better, even though early cosmetic improvement may please.

Sensibly used, steroid injections can also help inflamed hand joints and tendons, trigger fingers and nerve entrapments. Warm baths in wax or water soothe and allow gentle exercising. A range of gadgets and modified implements are available to extend the function of the rheumatoid hand and the occupational therapist can advise on these.

The Wrist

The wrist is the key to effective hand function because fixing the wrist in a position of slight extension is the prelude for most normal hand movements requiring any force. Since the wrist is often involved in rheumatoid, its preservation is important and steroid injections into the inflamed joint can be extremely effective in reducing pain and hence increasing function. The wrist need not be mobile to work well and since it is movement that causes pain, lightweight splints or surgical fusion of badly damaged wrists may improve hand function dramatically.

The Shoulders

Shoulders are commonly painful in rheumatoid and in the early stages injections help. In mechanically damaged shoulders, where pain is very severe and movement very limited, a replacement shoulder joint will give good pain relief but will not restore much movement. For this reason it is usually avoided while the natural joint retains reasonable mobility.

The Elbows

In most cases, elbow involvement must be borne stoically. Inflamed joints can be settled by the usual local and general treatments but, except in a few cases where part of the joint or the joint lining is removed, surgery has little place yet. Replacement joints so far have tended to have a short life and designs are constantly changing.

The Hip

The features of arthritis in the hip are described in Chapter 3. About a quarter of rheumatoid patients will develop it. Once pain is sufficiently severe, surgery should be offered to replace the joint.

The Knee

Preservation of the knee joint by drawing off effusions and injecting steroids, preserving the stabilising power of the quadriceps muscles by exercises, and splintage and physiotheraphy to straighten bent joints where possible, are all of extreme importance from early in the disease. Very unequal leg length will strain the knee on the longer side. The knee is also one of the commoner joints treated by surgical removal of the synovial lining, although the lining eventually does grow back. Knee joint replacement is increasingly used for the rheumatoid knee in the final stages of the disease.

Rheumatoid is the commonest arthritic condition in which the joint capsule swells out behind the knee to form a so-called Baker's cyst. This may rupture into the calf with pain, swelling and discoloration of the lower leg. Non-specialists usually diagnose phlebitis. The treatment is to put a support stocking on the leg and a steroid injection into the knee, when it will settle down over a week or so.

The Ankle

The hind foot has three joints, the ankle joint itself which waggles the foot up and down, the sub-talar joint immediately beneath it which allows sidewards movement of the ankle, and a collection of joints in the instep – the mid-tarsal joint. The commonest rheumatoid trouble in this region is for the sub-talar joint to be bent outwards so the patient walks on the inside edge of the foot. This causes strain and pain at the ankle and callouses and ulcers on the tender skin of the edge of the foot. The deformity can be corrected by subtle modifications to the sole and heel of the shoe, or by unobtrusive supporting devices, and the benefits in pain relief are often great.

Surgery to the ankle is not sophisticated. The usual operation is to stiffen all three joints (triple arthrodesis) in the correct alignment. Half measures just throw more wear on the other joints. Pain relief is excellent but since the joints take three months or so to fuse together completely there is a long post-operative period before full weight bearing is possible.

The Foot

Pain under the ball of the foot (metatarsalgia) is often the first symptom of rheumatoid arthritis. The common deformity in the advanced rheumatoid foot is for the toes to be bent upwards at the ball of the foot and to compensate, the next little joint in the toe bends downwards, producing a claw toe. Hallux valgus (*see* Chapter 3) is usually also present. These deformities produce callouses under the ball of the foot and at points where the shoes exert pressure. Good footwear, with moulded insoles to redistribute the weight, is very helpful. Patients with metatarsalgia, especially if they have mid-tarsal joint trouble as well, have no spring in their feet and shuffle along. A curved sole or a transverse bar behind the metatarsal heads may improve mobility. There are a number of surgical procedures to improve the rheumatoid foot. The surgeon will advise on the appropriate one in each case.

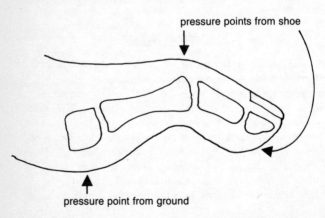

pressure points from shoe

pressure point from ground

Fig 12   Rheumatoid claw toe.

The Spine

For most of its length the spine has little to fear from rheumatoid arthritis. There can be inflammation of the discs, called discitis, but this does not usually give any bother. In the neck, however, the joints and ligaments between the top two vertebrae may be loosened, allowing excessive movement. The patient is often unaware of this but if it is painful a collar may be advised. The main concern is that the movement of head on neck may press on the spinal cord. Actually there is a lot of room in the spinal canal at

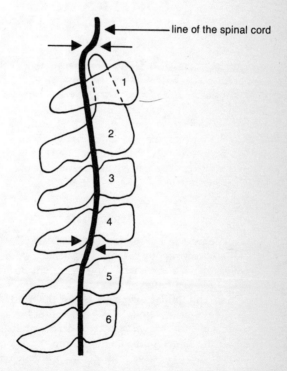

— line of the spinal cord

Fig 13 Instability in the rheumatoid spine. The first vertebra (atlas) has slipped forwards from the peg of the second vertebra and number 4 has slipped forwards on number 5.

this level and significant problems are unusual, but if they occur, surgical fusion may be needed.

The Jaw and Larynx

Involvement of the jaw joint is not uncommon and injections of steroid are very effective. The joints in the larynx move the vocal cords and may 'seize up', causing hoarseness and, at worst, hampering breathing, but this is a very, very rare occurrence.

COMPLICATIONS

Nodules

Nodules are a classical feature of rheumatoid arthritis but only occur in a quarter of patients. When present they denote sero-positive disease, usually with a greater tendency to erosions of joints, to vasculitis and other organ involvement. They form typically on pressure surfaces such as behind the elbow, or the back of the heel, but they may form internally and may be seen in the lungs on a chest X-ray, for example. They can be removed but will regrow and are not in themselves harmful, shrinking as the disease comes under control.

Vasculitis

Vasculitis means inflammation of blood vessels. There are very many different forms of vasculitis associated with many diseases and they range from trivial and transient to severe and life threatening. Fortunately vasculitis is a rare complication of rheumatoid and milder forms are by far the most common.

The commonest feature of rheumatoid vasculitis is the appearance of little brown specks of dead skin at the edge of the nails or in the finger pulp. These require no action though they imply the disease is active and so may influence decisions about therapy. More severe vasculitis can cause stubborn skin ulceration, or damage the gut or important nerves, and these more troublesome problems usually require treatment with steroids and immune-suppressing agents like cyclophosphamide or azathiaprine which can control even the more severe forms of vasculitis.

Amyloidosis

Active inflammatory disease produces substances circulating in the blood as mediators of the inflammatory process. Amyloidosis is the deposition of one of these substances which builds up in the tissues so that, with time, organ function may be disrupted. In rheumatoid disease the most important site of amyloid deposition is the kidneys and although progression may be very slow, some patients will eventually need treatment for kidney failure. There is no sure, direct treatment of amyloid itself, but its presence encourages increased efforts to control the rheumatoid inflammation.

Sjogren's Syndrome

Usually pronounced 'Shurr-gren's' syndrome, this condition may occur on its own, but it frequently co-exists with rheumatic diseases, especially rheumatoid arthritis. The underlying process is an auto-immune attack by lymphocytes on the lacrimal glands in the eyes which make tears, the salivary glands of the mouth and similar glands elsewhere. Patients notice gritty eyes and the loss of the protection of the tears leads to frequent conjunctivitis. Swallowing, especially of dry foods, is difficult and women may experience painful intercourse because of loss of vaginal secretions.

There is no 'cure'. Artificial tears are available and may be used as often as needed – carry a bottle with you. Operations to block the tear ducts may slow the rate at which tears drain from the eye. The dry mouth can only be managed by frequent drinks. Lubricants for the vagina may ease intercourse.

Felty's Syndrome

This is a rare condition of sero-positive rheumatoid patients where the numbers of white cells in the blood go down, increasing the risk of some infections. In practice, many patients seem to tolerate even very low white counts without serious trouble. The exact cause of this complication is unknown but in most cases the spleen is enlarged and its removal (splenectomy) will bring up the white cell numbers. This benefit may be transient, however, and there are risks of infection from splenectomy itself, so many rheumatologists prefer to avoid it if possible.

Involvement of other Organs

As well as Sjogren's syndrome, the eye can become inflamed as part of the rheumatoid disease itself. Most often this is merely a painless, reddened area in the white of the eye but more widespread, painful inflammation may require the same treatment as vasculitis.

I have already mentioned nodules in the lung but these do not usually produce symptoms. Rheumatoid patients also get attacks of pleurisy, a sharp pain in the chest made worse by coughing or sneezing, and sometimes quite large amounts of inflammatory fluid may collect in the chest (pleural effusion). Quite a number of rheumatoid patients have minor degrees of fibrosis in the lungs which never trouble them, but in a few the fibrosis slowly progresses to cause shortness of breath.

The fibrous sac surrounding the heart may also become inflamed (pericarditis). This may be without symptoms but can be heard as a rasping noise through the stethoscope. It can produce a similar sharp pain as pleurisy and indeed is essentially the same process at a different site. Less commonly, the sac may become persistently inflamed and thickened (chronic pericarditis) and limit the efficiency with which the heart pumps. Surgical removal of the thickened sac restores heart function to normal.

Although rheumatoid does not directly affect the skin, except as a consequence of vasculitis, the foot deformities and the skin-thinning effect of steroid therapy make skin ulceration a major feature of long-standing, severe rheumatoid. It is unsightly, depressing and exposes the patient to a range of infections. Long stays in hospital over months may be needed to heal a stubborn ulcer.

6

Polymyalgia Rheumatica

Polymyalgia rheumatica is a common illness of the elderly and very occasionally affects the middle-aged. It responds dramatically to treatment within a day or so. No one knows exactly what causes it but it is undoubtedly another immunological disorder.

The illness starts so suddenly that patients can often remember exactly what they were doing. The sufferer feels aching and pain, especially around the neck and shoulders and the low back, buttock and thighs. Symptoms are worse in the mornings and the patients feel ill in themselves and very often depressed. If they have had it for a while they may lose weight. Disability is severe. Sufferers usually cannot get out of chairs or the bath or climb stairs without great difficulty. Typically, they say that their partners push them out of bed in the morning.

Most patients show a moderate anaemia which we have already seen to be a common feature of generalised inflammatory disease. The ESR is very high (*see* Chapter 5). A very few patients just have abnormal blood tests, with a feeling of being ill and losing weight, without any clues that they have a rheumatic disease. They may undergo test after normal test until eventually the penny drops.

Once the penny has dropped, treatment is a moderate dose of steroid tablets and the patient is delighted, being back to normal within a day or so. Treatment is gradually reduced and after about two years the disease will usually blow out and the steroids can be stopped. A few patients do become ill again and have to be retreated for a while. Much more common, however, is the patient who thinks the disease has returned, but is actually feeling all the normal aches and pains of the elderly which were forgotten when on steroids.

Polymyalgia is not always as straightforward as this and a common problem is to distinguish it from rheumatoid arthritis, which sometimes starts in this way in the elderly. Since rheumatoid does not melt away easily with small doses of steroid we want to avoid the patient coming to depend on them. Sometimes, when uncertain, the doctor will give a trial of a small amount of steroid and if the results are dramatic he will be happier that the patient really has polymyalgia.

GIANT CELL ARTERITIS

Occasionally polymyalgia may accompany giant cell arteritis (also called cranial arteritis). Patients may have symptoms of both conditions at once or either may occur alone. Note that this is an *arteritis* not an arthritis, that is, an inflammation of the arteries and therefore one type of vasculitis (*see* Chapter 5). You may also hear it called temporal arteritis because the blood vessels running over the temples at the side of the head are often the ones where trouble is noticed.

The main symptom is a severe, constant headache. Not only that, but the scalp is tender so that brushing the hair or even wearing a hat may be unbearable. Occasionally the temples may be visibly swollen and inflamed. Temporal arteritis is a bad name, however, since many other blood vessels may be involved and patients may notice pain in the jaw when they eat or in the tongue when they speak because of cramp in the muscles whose blood flow is being cut off.

The vital importance of this illness is that the blood vessels to the eye are also involved, usually without the patient being aware of it, and sudden and irreversible blindness can occur. Steroids are started immediately on suspicion, using doses three or four times higher than in polymyalgia. The doctor may arrange a temporal artery biopsy – a little snip of the artery under local anaesthetic (it does no harm and you do not lose blood) and this sometimes shows the giant cells and confirms his suspicions. However, there are many patients where the decision to treat is made on the doctor's skilled opinion alone. Although the illness is more serious than polymyalgia, it responds just as rapidly.

7
Gout and Pseudogout

Everyone has heard of gout, but not many of pseudogout, yet they are both common conditions in which crystals form in the joint and generate inflammation. In each case this may produce a very painful, acute arthritis or more chronic joint damage.

GOUT

What is Gout?

Gout is due to the deposit of sodium urate salts in the tissues. Sodium urate is made in the liver as a breakdown product of chemicals called purines which are found in the nucleus of all cells. Urate is therefore made partly from the regular breakdown of our own worn-out tissues, and partly from the diet. The urate so formed circulates in the blood and is excreted in the urine. As blood levels of urate rise, there is an increasing chance that solid crystals of urate will be deposited in the tissues. This can cause two distinct arthritic conditions: acute gout and chronic, tophaceous gout.

Acute Gout

Sodium urate crystals form in the synovial lining of the joint and may be shed into the joint fluid where they are capable of triggering an intense inflammatory reaction resulting in an excruciatingly painful, tender arthritis. The first attacks are usually in a single joint, especially the big toe which suddenly becomes red, shiny and horribly sore, often in the middle of the night. The inflammation can be so florid that much of the limb may be swollen, red and painful and is often thought to be septic. Even without treatment, acute attacks of gout seem to switch themselves off in a week or so, but we do not know why. Some patients get attacks at long intervals but for many the attacks recur frequently involving several joints.

Chronic Tophaceous Gout

With continued high blood levels of urate over long periods cream-coloured lumps of solid urate can be seen overlying the knuckles and fingers, the tips of the ears or at those same pressure points which spawn rheumatoid nodules. These deposits are called tophi and may distend the skin to the point of ulceration, or if they develop in the joint, gross destructive changes may occur. Curiously, some people with chronic tophaceous gout do not have superimposed attacks of acute gout, but others do, often brought on by certain trigger situations (*see* pages 65–66). Prolonged tophaceous gout can lead to urate deposits in the kidneys, with eventual kidney failure, but with modern drugs this complication has virtually disappeared and chronic tophaceous gout itself is becoming a rarity.

Identifying Gout

Typical acute or tophaceous gout is obvious at a glance, yet, curiously, gout is often either missed or over-diagnosed. On the one hand, many are unaware that acute gout can attack several joints at once and so assume the patient has rheumatoid arthritis, especially if there are nodules on the elbows. On the other is the tendency to see a patient with an arthritis, find he has a high urate level in the blood and label him as having gout. High urate levels are common in men and they are as likely as anyone to have osteo-arthritis, especially at the great toe where a reddish bunion may form. Osteo-arthritis never produces the exquisite agony of gout, more a constant discomfort on weight bearing which is eased by rest, unlike gout. The only sure way of diagnosing gout is to extract some joint fluid and show the crystals under a microscope. Gout responds so well to correct treatment that if your drugs are not working, the diagnosis needs a rethink or you are not using them properly.

Treatment

It is important not to confuse the treatment for an acute attack of gout with the long-term preventive treatment. Acute gout should be treated as soon as possible with a high dose of an anti-inflammatory drug. Indomethacin is the most popular choice but any of this class will work and bring the attack under control within 48 hours. The drug is then taken in a lower dose for a week or so. Tablets should be easily available since gout strikes suddenly, and often at inconvenient times. If you are unable to take these drugs, for example, because of a stomach ulcer, then colchicine is just as good. It has a tendency to cause diarrhoea, hence the old rheumatological saying that it makes you 'run before you can walk'. Acute joints can also be injected with steroids, with rapid relief.

If attacks are frequent, or if you have tophaceous gout, preventive treatment should be used. This may be offered even if you have never had gout, if your blood urate is very high or if you have urate stones in your kidney. In most cases this treatment will be for life. The usual drug used is allopurinol, which blocks the production of urate so that eventually you get no more acute attacks and gradually the tophi dissolve away.

If allopurinol is started on its own, especially during an attack, it will actually begin by increasing the amount of urate passing into the joint from the shrinking deposits in the synovium, and can bring on frequent acute attacks. So, for the first three months an anti-inflammatory drug is given as well. Many patients (and sadly many doctors) do not appreciate this and treat acute attacks with short courses of allopurinol, with the miserable consequences of a vicious circle of continued acute gout. Not surprisingly the patients do not think much of the tablets and may go away untreated. There are other drugs which prevent gout by flushing the urate through the kidneys but these are not used so much these days. These drugs also need to be started with an anti-inflammatory tablet.

Who gets Gout?

Men have higher blood urate levels than women and are twenty times more likely to get gout, but levels rise in women after the menopause. About thirty per cent of patients have a family history.

Most people with high urate levels have a minor, probably inherited, kidney defect which slows urate excretion. People with severe kidney disease have very high urate levels yet curiously many never suffer gout.

Doctors are themselves responsible for gout in some patients since diuretics (water tablets) can causes rises in blood urate. Taking one aspirin tablet every other day is quite widely used nowadays in the hope of reducing heart disease and strokes, and this will also increase the urate level.

The traditional gout sufferer is thought to be one who over-indulges in rich food and alcohol, especially those with a high purine content such as liver, fish and strong beers or wines. However, we now believe that it is not the purine content of the diet that is so important but the fact that obesity results in high urate levels and alcohol raises these further by effects on production and excretion.

Managing Gout

Since modern drug treatment is so good, you could almost be advised to 'keep taking the tablets and enjoy yourself'. However, you would be well advised to lose weight (but not rapidly, as that may precipitate gout) and cut down on alcohol. Unaccustomed exercise may also induce gout, so it is not all bad news.

PSEUDOGOUT

This is almost exclusively a disease of the elderly, affecting women more often than men, and is very common but little known to the public. It is due to the deposit of calcium pyrophosphate salts in the joint tissues, especially the cartilage, but unlike sodium urate it is not deposited anywhere else. This calcification can be seen on the X-ray and becomes increasingly common with age. Many of these people will also have osteo-arthritic changes. Calcium pyrophosphate is more likely to deposit in a damaged joint and a very small number of people may have an underlying fault in the body chemistry. For over 90 per cent of people, however, joint calcification is just a feature of aging.

Not all people with calcium on the X-ray will have trouble with their joints, but if calcium pyrophosphate crystals are shed into the joint, they can generate a severe acute arthritis with exactly the same florid appearance and pain as gout, hence the name. Such attacks may come on without obvious reason but they often follow injury to the joint or any surgery. The distinction of pseudogout from gout is made by drawing off the fluid and recognising the differently shaped crystals.

Just as gout has a chronic form, so does pseudogout, but there are no tophi. The patient usually has pain in a few joints, especially the knees. The picture is like a fairly severe form of osteo-arthritis. Unlike simple osteo-arthritis, chronic pseudogout produces more inflammatory changes in the joints, which become more damaged.

A florid crystal arthritis, be it gout or pseudogout, may produce a nasty, feverish illness and may be mistaken for infection. Elderly people can be quite confused and unwell during this period, but return to normal when the pain is eased.

The treatment of acute pseudogout is just like the treatment of acute gout, except that colchicine is not effective. There is no preventive treatment for pseudogout like allopurinol for gout. In both conditions a badly damaged joint should be considered for surgical replacement, just as in any other arthritis. You do not have to worry about diet or alcohol with pseudogout, although it is sensible to keep your weight down.

SEPTIC ARTHRITIS

Septic arthritis implies a bacterial infection within a joint and usually occurs having spread via the bloodstream from an infection elsewhere in the body, such as pneumonia. Usually only one joint is affected and the arthritis is often exceedingly florid and tender, as in gout. Joints already damaged by other forms of arthritis are especially at risk and may be mistaken for a flare of the disease, but anyone with a single *suddenly very inflamed* joint, or those with arthritis where one joint begins acting out of character with the others, should consult their doctor.

Most of the common bacteria can infect joints. Untreated septic arthritis will destroy the joint and can kill. Infection is diagnosed by drawing off some of the joint fluid and detecting the bacteria. Treatment is with antibodies over several weeks.

Long-standing septic arthritis is usually less obvious and is rare. Tuberculosis and the unfortunate infection of an artificial joint are the main causes.

8

Ankylosing Spondylitis and Related Disorders

This family of disorders has some features in common. They tend to attack large joints, although small joints may be involved, and all can involve the spine and sacro-iliac joints, although this is only common in ankylosing spondylitis. They may also share similar, non-arthritic complications.

ANKYLOSING SPONDYLITIS

This is not particularly common and most sufferers are men. We now think that the condition occurs nearly as often in women but usually in so mild a form that they rarely notice it.

Spondylitis means inflammation of the spine and should not be confused with *spondylosis* – the term used for the degenerative changes seen on X-ray which we all get as we grow older (*see* Chapter 4). The inflammatory process begins in the sacro-iliac joints (sacroiliitis), at the junction of the lowest spinal vertebrae and the iliac bones of the pelvis. Inflammation also develops where the vertebral bodies are attached to the fibrous capsule of the disc. Calcium salts are deposited in these inflamed areas and gradually form bony spurs (syndesmophytes) which grow out to meet similar spurs from adjacent vertebrae (*see* Fig 14). If the disease is neglected these spurs may eventually meet and fuse the vertebrae together over a greater or lesser extent of the spine. The facet joints can also fuse so the spine may become very stiff. The sacro-iliac joints also become welded together with time, but since they are not normally required to move much anyway, this is no great loss. Such bony fusion is called ankylosis (hence ankylosing spondylitis) but nowadays extensive fusion of the spine is most unusual in well-managed patients.

The early symptoms of ankylosing spondylitis will usually begin in young men with pain across the low back, buttocks and thighs just as in lumbago. Of course, most young men with backache will have non-specific mechanical back pain, not ankylosing spondylitis, and there are characteristic differences. Ankylosing spondylitis tends to be gradual and persistent, it is eased by exercise and worse after resting, with prolonged morning stiffness and aching typical of inflammatory disease, all in contrast to the usual forms of back ache.

The condition does not only affect the spine and the first symptoms may be an inflammatory arthritis of one, or a few, large limb joints, especially hip, knee or shoulder. Some very rare patients even have a distribution of arthritis just like rheumatoid. The tendency to attack the junction between bones and capsules or ligaments, as in the spine, also occurs elsewhere and chest pain is a frequent complaint due to tenderness at the junction of rib muscles and the skeleton. Similarly, plantar fasciitis, achilles tendonitis and related conditions are all more common in ankylosing spondylitis.

Since it is a generalised inflammatory condition, active ankylosing spondylitis makes sufferers tired and unwell. A few are anaemic and some really feel quite ill. There are other non-arthritic features, notably iritis, a painful inflammation of the eye which affects about one-third of patients. Usually the doctor can decide on a diagnosis from the pattern of the illness, plus simple X-rays, but he may arrange an isotope scan to show up sacroiliitis not yet visible on X-ray.

The Outlook for the Disease

Nearly all patients with ankylosing spondylitis live normal working lives to retirement. For some, pain eases after a few years and they simply go through life with a stiff lumbosacral spine – no great hardship. In those where active phases persist or recur and spinal disease is more extensive, good posture and movement can be maintained by regular exercises. The textbooks show pictures of bent old men, their eyes permanently looking to the ground, and this is what your family doctor may remember. However, such cases are now virtually never seen except in those who have neglected their disease.

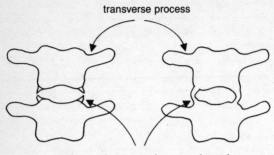

transverse process

syndesmophytes growing towards each
other and fusing

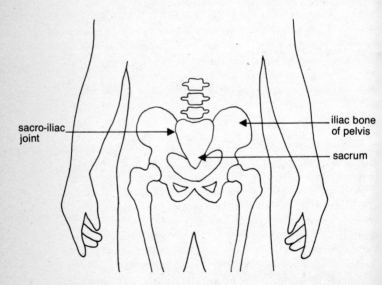

sacro-iliac
joint

iliac bone
of pelvis

sacrum

Fig 14   Spinal changes in ankylosing spondylitis.

Treatment

The first essential is to emphasise the optimistic outlook for the patient and encourage him to perform a regular exercise programme daily. This should be simple and quick. Specifically, the back should be bent backwards to its limit, bent sideways, and rotated in each direction, followed by full extension and rotation of the neck and the movements are then repeated at least a dozen times. If you wish to do more, concentrate on general physical fitness; swimming is perfect. Some insist on breathing exercises, telling you that without them your chest will eventually become too stiff to breathe. This is frightening and not true. Finally, it is helpful to have a firm bed and to spend at least twenty minutes each day lying flat on your face to correct any tendency to bend forward.

The stiffness of ankylosing spondylitis is usually helped by anti-inflammatory tablets, especially phenylbutazone which is now used only for this condition, although most prefer to start with indomethacin because of restrictions on phenylbutazone (*see* Chapter 10). This sort of treatment also helps the joints and their general management is just the same as in any other inflammatory arthritis. The limb joints can benefit from gold or penicillamine 'second line' treatment, as in rheumatoid, but these drugs do not seem to help the spine. Recent trials suggest sulphasalazine may help joints and spine. Very severely unwell patients may be given steroids and other immuno-suppressive agents. The complication of iritis must have prompt treatment with steroid drops and sometimes tablets for a while.

Causes

Of white people who have ankylosing spondylitis, 95 per cent carry the gene HLA B27. This is not one of the HLA genes which influence interactions between cells of the immune system, like HLA DR4 found in some patients with rheumatoid arthritis, so we cannot explain the association in the same way as we can in that case.

Reiter's syndrome (*see* page 72) also has a very close link with HLA B27 and we know that disease often follows infections of the bowel. There is some experimental work suggesting that Klebsiella, a bacterium that can involve the gut, may trigger ankylosing spondylitis, although not everyone believes this. One mechanism might be that the antigenic structure of Klebsiella and the gene HLA B27 are similar, so that antibodies made against Klebsiella may attack host cells carrying HLA B27.

You may think it odd that doctors do not test everyone with back pain for HLA B27, but 80 per cent of people with HLA B27 have nothing wrong with them, so its presence does not mean you have ankylosing spondylitis.

REITER'S SYNDROME

In this condition an arthritis affecting a few large joints can be seen to be related to a preceding infection and thus it is often called reactive arthritis. The infection is either non-specific urethritis (NSU) which is a venereal disease, or else some form of infective diarrhoea. Up to 90 per cent of sufferers will have the HLA B27 gene.

Some time within about three months from infection a very tender arthritis begins, typically in the knee or ankle, often with all the florid inflammatory features seen in gout or sepsis. Usually only a few large joints become involved, but some patients develop a more generalised arthritis, including small joints in hands or feet. Single toes or fingers may become swollen along their length like sausages.

The arthritis will be accompanied by non-arthritic features such as conjunctivitis, ulcers in the mouth or a ring of florid, painless ulcers around the tip of the penis like a 'ring of roses'. There may be a discharge from the penis even in those without VD and scaly rashes may affect the soles or palms which are indistinguishable from certain forms of psoriasis. Even when an infective trigger cannot be established these characteristic features allow the diagnosis to be made and on this basis it is probably the commonest arthritis of young adults.

It used to be taught that the arthritis nearly always cleared up within a few months, but probably 60 per cent have intermittent or persistent symptoms over a longer period. About a third of these will get the spinal changes of ankylosing spondylitis and quite a few get iritis, illustrating the overlap which can occur in this family of disorders. The short-lived form of Reiter's is usually easy to control with conventional measures of rest, splintage, joint injection and anti-inflammatory drugs. Treatment of any venereal infection may be needed in its own right, together with advice about sexual hygiene and tracing of contacts, but treatment of venereal or bowel infection will not alter the course of the arthritis.

By contrast, persistent Reiter's disease can be quite difficult to treat satisfactorily. Non-specific measures help but there is no accepted form of second line treatment. The usual agents are tried in severe cases and sulphasalazine and methotrexate hold some promise.

Diarrhoea or VD?

Many doctors still think of Reiter's syndrome as invariably a product of venereal infection and they provoke guilt, embarrassment or, more properly, anger in many patients. I have never seen why catching a venereal disease should be frowned upon, although passing one on is a different matter. In any case, we now feel that very many attacks are not venereal but due to bowel infections, some so mild as to go unnoticed. The fact that the patient has a urethral discharge does not mean they have a venereal disease, although it would be foolish not to check. Such a discharge is a part of Reiter's syndrome, however initiated.

PSORIATIC ARTHRITIS

Psoriasis is a very common skin disorder in which about 8 per cent of patients have some form of arthritis. Most people with psoriatic arthritis have a much milder disease than rheumatoid. Some patients may not know they have psoriasis and show no sign of it or only very subtle areas in out of the way places such as the scalp, navel, nails or between the buttocks. So now you know what the doctor was looking for!

There are different patterns of psoriatic arthritis. In about three-quarters of patients it concentrates on a few large joints or may affect joints of the hands in a more random asymmetrical distribution than rheumatoid. A second group have an arthritis that looks just like rheumatoid arthritis but is milder and without nodules or the other non-arthritic complications of rheumatoid disease. A small minority of patients have a disease like ankylosing spondylitis. Finally, there is a tiny number of unfortunates with a rapidly destructive form of the disease called arthritis mutilans. Unfortunately, many think this is the only form of psoriatic arthritis, whereas it is actually exceedingly rare.

Treatment for simple disease is exactly what you will now have come to expect for inflammatory arthritis. Second line drugs used in rheumatoid have been successfully extended to psoriatic arthritis, but some patients find chloroquine worsens their skin disease. Treatment of the skin generally makes little impact on the arthritis but some severe forms of skin disease are treated with immuno-suppressive drugs and these will, of course, exert an effect on inflamed joints. One of these agents, Methotrexate, has been so effective for joints that it is now being used successfully in severe cases of rheumatoid arthritis and Reiter's syndrome.

INFLAMMATORY BOWEL DISEASE

This includes Crohn's disease and ulcerative colitis, two uncommon conditions which may be complicated by a relatively mild arthritis of a few large joints, or a spondylitis, and so form a fourth member of the family. Because of their similarity in many features some patients thought to have Reiter's syndrome, whose diarrhoea persists, may turn out to be cases of inflammatory bowel disease.

FAMILY MATTERS

Because they share a genetic susceptibility, these arthritic conditions tend to crop up in families but the number of affected members is very small so you should not be afraid of getting arthritis or passing it on to a child just because a relative has such a disease.

9
Coping with Arthritis

Many people with rheumatic complaints will have no reason to consult a doctor because they either recover spontaneously or never have sufficient discomfort or disability to let it worry them. Others will manage with occasional pain-killers and by common-sense adjustments to life-style, clothing or footwear. However, if your activities are annoyingly limited, if you are worrying about getting worse, or your joints remain painfully inflamed, you would be wise to see a doctor. The majority who attend a rheumatology clinic will receive a reassuring diagnosis of osteo-arthritis or a non-arthritic, rheumatic condition. No treatment may be needed apart from revealing the favourable outcome, answering questions and giving simple advice. Once uncertainty is removed, many people can cope with pain which they previously found intolerable. Some will benefit from local steroid injections, physiotherapy or simple appliances. Drugs will be limited to simple pain-killers or anti-inflammatory agents. Since these only treat symptoms, you can do without them if you prefer.

For those with a truly inflammatory arthritis several visits may go by without a firm diagnosis, while the rheumatologist watches the pattern of the illness. You should not be alarmed by this; many arthritic conditions look similar in their early stages and all are initially managed on the same non-specific lines as above. There is nothing to show that the long-term outlook is improved by beginning specific treatments at the earliest possible moment. These treatments carry risks and tie you closer to the clinic, so it is nice if they can be avoided, especially since some very florid arthritic illnesses clear up over a few weeks and months without a diagnosis being made. This is a frustrating time, of course, especially if your symptoms are not adequately controlled and at some stage the doctor may feel it necessary to add one of the more specific treatments on the basis of a definite or probable diagnosis and on an assessment of disease activity (*see* Chapter 5).

At different times you may be referred to other specialists:

physiotherapists, occupational therapists, social workers, chiropodists or surgical fitters. However, most of the time you will be coping yourself, at home and at work.

GENERAL HEALTH

Exercise or Rest?

Patients are often unclear whether they should exercise or rest. Acutely tender joints should be rested, but immobility stiffens inflamed joints so they should be rested in a position which preserves function even if the joint were to become restricted. Knees should be straight – you must not put a pillow behind them, no matter how comfortable. Bent knees limit walking considerably and accelerate joint damage. Wrists should not droop but be slightly extended and bedclothes should not weigh the foot down at the ankle – use a bed cradle. Maintaining a functional position over long periods in bed may require splints.

Joints that are not acutely tender should be used within the limits of mild discomfort. There is no benefit in pushing beyond the pain barrier. If you have been resting in hospital, return to full activity will be supervised by a physiotherapist, often using the warmth and buoyancy of the hydrotherapy pool. As well as increasing movement you will need to rebuild wasted muscles. Many rheumatologists like patients to perform a daily exercise programme, putting all their joints through their maximum range of pain-free movement. However, I prefer to encourage general exercise up to whatever level you can achieve.

Basically, the arthritic patient cannot 'do too much' but should follow activity by adequate rest. When inflammatory activity is intense, the whole body will need rest, sometimes in hospital, and even when the disease is fairly quiet, rheumatoid patients should set aside regular rest periods during the day.

Alcohol and Smoking

Alcohol, in moderate amounts, is cheering, relaxing and a mild pain reliever – there is no reason why you should not enjoy it in any form you like. There are no anti-rheumatic drugs which cannot be taken with alcohol but in immoderate amounts it acts as a gastric irritant and is potentially harmful in conjunction with irritant drugs such as steroids or anti-inflammatory agents. Co-proxamole (distalgesic) and muscle relaxant drugs have a sedative effect which is exaggerated by alcohol, but I am not in favour of the absolute avoidance of alcohol as directed by the pharmacy.

There are many reasons for not smoking, but arthritis is not one of them.

WORK AND ARTHRITIS

Many patients attribute their arthritis to their type of work. Such connections are difficult to establish but are probably true for some soft-tissue rheumatism. Inappropriate trauma to a joint will predispose to osteo-arthritis but it is not felt that normal use harms joints no matter how repetitive; it may even protect them. None of the inflammatory diseases in this book is connected with particular occupations.

A small number of seriously affected patients will not be able to continue their usual work or will need long periods off work. Generally it is wiser to tell your employer and put them in touch with your consultant. They may be prepared to allow you time off if the future outlook is good and, if not, they will be better placed to find you realistic alternative work. If you lose your job, you may be helped by the Disability Resettlement Officer, contactable through the Job Centre or hospital.

DAY-TO-DAY LIVING

Clothing

Loss of manual dexterity and restricted movement at large joints may make dressing difficult or impossible. Independence can be maintained by choosing clothing with an eye to the ease of getting it on and off and by replacing buttons, zips or shoe-laces with velcro straps. Ties can be pre-knotted and put on elastic and there are gadgets to help with socks and stockings. The occupational therapist advises on these and they can be viewed along with other home equipment in the Disabled Living Foundation showrooms around the country.

Footwear is very important for most arthritics. Shoes should be broad, deep enough not to rub and have a thick sole to cushion the ground. Low heels offer more stability and do not throw your weight on to the often painful balls of the feet. The Arthritis and Rheumatism Council (ARC) produces an excellent pamphlet on choosing shoes and chiropodists are very knowledgeable in caring for arthritic feet.

Personal Toilet

The same disabilities which lead to difficulties with clothing also make it hard to brush your hair, bath or go to the lavatory. Difficulties in these important and personal areas should be reported to your doctor if he does not ask. Most patients with significant disability will be assessed by the occupational therapist in what is termed ADL (Aids to Daily Living), to identify such difficulties as well as problems with day-to-day housework, cooking, dressing, etc. They can advise on the wide number of often superb gadgets designed to help you.

About the Home

I am not going to list ideas for reorganising the different rooms of the house, nor the innumerable devices that can help with household tasks. Everyone has their own individual needs, and equipment which is foisted on the disabled is rarely used. Far better be assessed in your home by the occupational therapist who has an eagle eye for difficulties and a fund of solutions. You can also see equipment in your local Disabled Living Foundation showroom and the ARC produce a booklet called *Aids and Gadgets in the Home*.

Getting About

Physiotherapists can achieve miracles of mobilisation in patients who have been virtually chair-bound, by building up confidence and muscle power and teaching how to distribute weight more effectively. Sticks and a variety of crutches or walking frames can be provided if necessary.

For many people, the wheelchair is the badge of disability and patients tend either to fall into one too soon, and rapidly lose independence, or are too reluctant at the time when a wheelchair would extend their mobility significantly. The NHS can provide wheelchairs but at present the only electrically propelled ones available on prescription are indoor chairs. Wheelchairs are provided by limb-fitting centres on prescription from your GP or specialist, or you can buy more elaborate models privately, but I would strongly advise anyone thinking of getting a chair to discuss it with a rheumatologist first: you may need a hip replacement.

All arthritic patients should drive if possible. You may be entitled to a mobility allowance from the DHSS which can then be used towards purchase or lease of a car (or outdoor electric chair) through the Motability scheme. The Royal Association for Disability and Rehabilitation (RADAR) provides a guide to choosing and modifying cars and the British School of Motoring have an assessment and training centre. The orange badge allowing unrestricted parking has been selfishly abused, but you can still get one if, in medical opinion, you cannot walk fifty yards. Public transport still poses problems but you can often get information and help on longer journeys if you contact the relevant company or authority. The Department of Environment issues a useful booklet on public transport for the disabled, *Door to Door*.

Sexual Activity

The effects of chronic ill health, diminished self-esteem and the depression that can accompany a nasty arthritis will reduce sexual drive. Together with problems imposed by painful, unyielding joints, the result is that for many, sexual activity stops. Many find the affection between partners sufficient but without a sexual dimension some relationships suffer and the arthritic sufferer loses a morale-boosting activity. Sexual Problems of the Disabled (SPOD) is one of a few agencies supplying counselling and it also produces a booklet. Much of this is common sense but some need reassurance to experiment with their sex life.

Contraception and Pregnancy

Arthritis may make barrier contraception difficult but your partner may enjoy helping. Although the contraceptive pill can occasionally cause aching joints and may adversely affect the rare rheumatic disease SLE, it can be used in rheumatoid and other forms of arthritis.

Very ill women do not get pregnant easily, but there is no reason why an arthritic patient should not plan a family. There are no common arthritic conditions for which the risk of handing on the disease need worry you.

Low back pain is a common problem in pregnancy and so is carpal tunnel syndrome. Rheumatoid arthritis virtually always improves dramatically during pregnancy but may recur a few weeks after birth. Other inflammatory conditions are less predictable and a minority of patients with SLE may get worse, although this should not discourage them from having children. SLE is also associated with a slightly higher rate of foetal loss, but modern combined medical and obstetric care means that most will have a healthy baby. Drugs in pregnancy and breast feeding are considered in Chapter 10.

Leisure and Social Life

Ideally, your social and leisure activities will be unchanged but you may need to think of new ways of doing things or of new things to do. I doubt if there is a single activity that some disabled person somewhere is not doing, so I do not see the value in a list of suggestions and possibilities. Most activities have their own governing bodies or enthusiasts' clubs and nearly all provide information for the disabled, often in printed form. The Disabled Living Foundation and RADAR have access to piles of information on activities, transport, accommodation access, etc.

See Useful Addresses for those of the more prominent organisations offering help. They can put you in touch with others.

10
Drugs and Treatment

SELECTING DRUGS

Patients expect their drugs to benefit them and not carry side-effects. At first sight this is not unreasonable, yet many find a tablet does not help and they are increasingly aware how many medical problems are due to drug side-effects. Encouraged by an ill-informed press to regard the occurrence of a side-effect as an error, the doctor is naturally seen as responsible. Patients become more and more reluctant to accept our treatments and they turn to what they see as safer, alternative therapies (*see* Chapter 11).

There is always an element of chance in prescribing a drug for an individual. When a new drug has finished its lengthy laboratory development, it is tried out on large numbers of volunteer patients. These trials are rigorously designed to ensure fair play and the results are further criticised in the medical press to uncover any features which might have biased the outcome. All patients selected must have the condition the drug claims to treat. This may seem terribly obvious but many arthritic diseases are hard to tell apart and a pill which helped 90 per cent of patients with a rag-bag of conditions might not do so well if used exclusively for rheumatoid arthritis. Suitable patients are then divided into two or more groups made up to be as nearly as possible identical in terms of disease severity, age, sex, etc. The new pill is given to one group and compared with either a dummy tablet (placebo) or the current standard treatments given to the other group or groups. After a while the groups cross over their treatments. The patients will not know when they are taking the dummy and when the real pills; we say they are 'blind'. To make things even fairer, the doctor recording their progess and the incidence of side-effects is also 'blind'. Treatment is chosen at random for each patient by another doctor who will reveal who has taken what at the end of the study.

Very few drugs will approach 100 per cent effectiveness, even if tolerated. Presumably this variability in response is partly due to differences in disease severity and partly to the present lack of knowledge about subtle variations within a single condition. It is, however, mainly because we are rarely treating the root causes. The more we understand the fundamental processes underlying a disease, the better we can design drugs and the greater the percentage who will respond. Antibiotics, therefore, approach or achieve 100 per cent effectiveness, whereas any anti-rheumatic drug rarely benefits more than 70 per cent of patients.

No drug will be free of side-effects because they are designed to interfere with metabolic processes and there are genetic differences in metabolism between individuals. They are also foreign materials and so a minority of patients will be allergic to them (note that this is not because they are unnatural; pollen is natural, but people are still allergic to it). A drug will be accepted for use if its side-effects are felt to be either sufficiently rare or non-serious to make the risk of taking the drug a reasonable one. Obviously, the judgement of risk will vary with the severity of the illness the drug has to treat.

So, you can be sure the drug works for your condition but not necessarily for you, and we cannot guarantee that there will be no side-effects. In this situation your idea of acceptable risk will differ from mine and from that of other patients. I think doctors should take patients into their confidence over such uncertainties and allow them to enter into the decision-making so that treatments are begun as an informal contract in good faith.

ANTI-INFLAMMATORY DRUGS

These are the main treatment for arthritic symptoms. They have pain-killing (analgesic) properties but also anti-inflammatory effects, seen at their most dramatic in the rapid relief of acute gout. They also ease the stiffness and aching characteristic of rheumatoid or ankylosing spondylitis. In non-inflammatory conditions or 'burnt-out' rheumatoid their analgesic properties may be helpful, but simple pain-killers are often as effective and probably safer.

Much of their action is due to their inhibition of enzymes on the chain of chemical reactions which produces inflammatory mediators called prostaglandins. Other important pathways are not blocked, which is probably why their anti-inflammatory effect is limited.

Common side-effects are rashes, sickness, diarrhoea and sometimes headaches. In the elderly they may occasionally cause total confusion. They can, in rare cases, worsen symptoms of some asthmatics.

Their most important side-effect is a tendency to irritate or ulcerate the lining of the stomach, mainly due to inhibition of a prostaglandin which protects the stomach lining. Attempts to reduce this effect, by giving the drug by suppository or designing it to be absorbed after it has passed through the stomach, do not work because much of the prostaglandin inhibition takes place in the bloodstream after the drug has been absorbed.

Kidney function is slightly reduced with a tendency to salt and water retention. This is usually of little consequence but occasionally swollen ankles may occur and, in the elderly, the heart and circulation may become overloaded. Very rarely, inflammatory disease of the kidney can occur (interstitial nephritis or nephrotic syndrome). Like all anti-inflammatory drug effects these kidney problems are reversible. Patients taking anti-coagulant tablets to thin the blood should not take anti-inflammatory tablets because they increase the risk of bleeding if the dosage of the anti-coagulant is not adjusted. There are occasions when it may be necessary, but careful monitoring will be vital.

Aspirin in high dose (twelve or more tablets per day) was the original anti-inflammatory drug. None of the many newer ones is more effective, but may have the convenience of requiring less frequent dosage or having greater tolerability. Some of these are: Azapropazone, Benorylate, Diclofenac, Diflunisal, Etodolac, Fenbufen, Fenopron, Flurbiprofen, Ibuprofen, Indomethacin, Ketoprofen, Mefenamic Acid, Nabumetone, Naproxen (Phenylbutazone), Piroxicam, Sulindac, Tiaprofenic Acid, Tolmetin. These are generic names. Some products, especially Aspirin, Ibuprofen and Indomethacin, have more than one trade name and this may be what your doctor uses when he prescribes. If you cannot see your anti-inflammatory here, ask your doctor or look for the generic name which will be on the packet.

Patients show definite personal preferences for different members of this group of drugs, so several should be tried to find the most suitable. Because inflammatory symptoms worsen over-night, it is usual to take one dose at bedtime and one on rising, but you should adjust your own timing to get the greatest benefit. You should take them with at least a milky drink or snack.

Anti-inflammatory drugs are often in the front line of media attention because such large numbers are consumed that the total number of adverse reactions is bound to be large. They are over-prescribed for conditions where simple analgesics do as well, but they are a really valuable class of drug which relieves much suffer-ing. Note that one of them, Ibuprofen, is available without prescription.

Phenylbutazone

This anti-inflammatory is now only available from hospitals for use in ankylosing spondylitis where it seems especially effective. It car-ries a very rare side-effect of bone marrow toxicity which makes it inappropriate for indiscriminate use.

SIMPLE ANALGESICS

Paracetamol, codeine, low-dose aspirin and some newer drugs are simply pain-killers. They are useful on their own or with anti-inflammatory agents. Certain tablets combine an analgesic with a relaxant such as Co-proxamole (distalgesic) containing paracetamol and dextropropoxyphene. It is no stronger than paracetamol alone and the preference many patients have for it is probably due to its habit-forming relaxant properties. Dex-tropropoxyphene is also very dangerous in overdose. However, used sensibly, many patients swear by 'DG' and many doctors reluctantly prescribe them.

SECOND LINE DRUGS

Anti-inflammatory drugs are rarely completely effective in severe rheumatoid arthritis and a second line of therapy is added, using slower-acting drugs with much more profound anti-inflammatory effects – they are often considered to modify the actual disease process. Not every rheumatologist believes this, but they are certainly very effective and have been extended to treat psoriatic arthritis, ankylosing spondylitis and some other inflammatory arthritic diseases. They are not used in osteo-arthritis. These drugs all have the potential for serious toxicity, so a decision to use them needs careful thought, but with close monitoring they actually prove remarkably safe in practice. We do not know for certain how any of them work.

Chloroquine

This anti-malarial drug is probably the weakest but also the safest of the second line drugs. It can cause rashes or stomach upsets but its only serious side-effect is retinal damage in high dose. With modern dosage this fear is largely unjustified and regular eye checks are carried out to get early warning of trouble.

Gold

Precious metals have been valued in medicine for centuries without scientific basis, but a major trial in the 1960s showed the benefit of gold. About a quarter of patients will be unable to tolerate gold, but side-effects are reversible and with good monitoring serious consequences are exceedingly uncommon. I divide side-effects into three groups: those the patient may notice, such as itchy rash or mouth ulcers; those the doctor will look out for with blood and urine tests, such as inflammation of the kidney or reduced production of white cells and platelets in the blood; and thirdly a number of exceedingly rare complications which I will not list in detail. This is to prevent patients becoming introspective about things which are unlikely to happen and I would simply encourage them to report any unusual happenings.

A gold compound is given by intramuscular injection every week and benefit may not appear for three months or so, at which time injections are reduced to once a month and are continued indefinitely. If there has been no improvement after a reasonable total dose of gold, it is considered to have failed. Side-effects may appear at any stage, so urine and blood checks are made with each injection. Only about 60 per cent of patients have long-term benefit from gold, but that still represents considerable relief of misery.

A tablet form of gold is now available (Auranofin). It is rather less effective but also less toxic.

Penicillamine

Treatment is begun with a 125mg tablet daily and the dose is increased by this amount every month until benefit is achieved or side-effects intervene. Few patients need more than 500mg daily, but there are no hard and fast rules. The main side-effects are very similar to those of gold, but there is a different list of very rare complications. As with gold, about 60 per cent benefit and blood and urine is checked monthly. Penicillamine should never be taken at the same time of day as iron tablets since neither would be absorbed.

Sulphasalazine

This drug is a mainstay of treatment for inflammatory bowel disease, but recently it has been shown to be an effective second line drug for rheumatoid arthritis and conditions such as ankylosing spondylitis which are related to inflammatory bowel disorders (*see* Chapter 8). About 20 per cent of patients experience side-effects, mostly mild and all reversible. Nausea or diarrhoea are the most common and rashes are not infrequent. Rapidly reversible male sterility may occur. Sulphasalazine can cause anaemia by damaging red blood cells and very rarely it suppresses the formation of white blood cells, so frequent blood checks are needed at first, then every few months.

IMMUNE-SUPPRESSING DRUGS

This class includes azathioprine, methotrexate, cyclophosphamide and others less often used. All are capable of serious toxicity and were originally used for cancer where high risks were thought justified. Experience and lower dosage has allowed their safe use in non-malignant conditions including inflammatory arthritis. Mild nausea is common and hair loss may occur.

Cyclophosphamide irritates the bladder and you should drink at least six pints of fluid per day when taking that drug. Methotrexate can damage the liver but this does not seem to be a major problem in the doses used for arthritis. The major side-effect of all these drugs is suppression of the bone marrow and immune system with consequent risks of bleeding or serious infection if treatment is not supervised. Although there is a theoretical risk that immune suppression increases the risks of developing malignant diseases, there is evidence that this is not so for arthritic patients treated with the commoner of these drugs. Even so, we restrict their use in younger patients.

Although all this sounds alarming, in practice problems are rare. These drugs are well tolerated and certainly work very effectively; in some situations they are life saving.

STEROIDS

Steroids are chemicals sharing a common ring structure. Some occur naturally, others are made synthetically. Although 'sex steroids' and 'anabolic steroids' are related compounds, they have nothing to do with the treatment of arthritis. Cortisone is a steroid produced naturally in the adrenal gland and has a host of vital functions: controlling body water and salt content, blood pressure, blood sugar, growth and bone formation. It also has the capacity to suppress many features of the inflammatory response. The production of cortisone fluctuates during twenty-four hours, being reduced overnight, and this may be why rheumatoid patients feel worse at night. Physical stress causes a major rise in steroid output. The influence of steroids is so widespread that without them we die.

With the development of synthetic steroids, substances were produced with anti-inflammatory effects many times greater than natural steroids and they were soon tried in rheumatoid arthritis. In high dosage the effects on inflammation were dramatic, and symptomatic improvement could be virtually complete. Unfortunately, these powerful drugs retained the other actions of cortisone so that it became apparent that patients taking steroids over long periods ran increased risks of diabetes, high blood pressure, heart disease and stroke, thinning and ulceration of the skin, loss of bone (osteoporosis), bloating and hairyness of face and trunk. There is also a significant risk of serious infections especially when combined with other immune-suppressants. Patients regularly using doses above the amount normally produced by their own adrenal gland would suppress their adrenal activity completely, so that if the tablets were stopped suddenly, or the patient underwent physical stress such as trauma or infection, he would be unable to produce a steroid response and might die.

Set alongside the toll of adverse effects was the observation that although rheumatoid symptoms improved, there was little evidence that the disease stopped damaging joints. Most rheumatologists now reserve steroids for situations requiring a rapid symptomatic response in a very ill patient who needs to get back to work or family. They are also justified in very elderly patients or where life-threatening complications arise, such as vasculitis. Patients on steroids should carry a card to say so until about two years after they have come off them and they should never stop or reduce treatment without medical approval.

Injecting Steroids into Joints

Steroids injected into soft tissues or joints stay at the site of injection to produce a prolonged local anti-inflammatory effect without the risk of long-term adverse reactions. A little does seep into the blood to give a brief general 'buzz' of well-being and diabetics may notice they pass a bit more sugar in the urine for a few days. We restrict the number of injections made into weight-bearing joints although there is no proof that they harm human joints used this way. They are much more effective in actively inflamed joints than in osteo-arthritis.

DRUGS IN PREGNANCY AND BREAST-FEEDING

The general rule that all drugs are best avoided in pregnancy should be applied. Rheumatoid arthritis rarely needs treatment in pregnancy, anyway. However, women will be worried about becoming pregnant while on treatment, yet reluctant to stop drugs, since successful conception may take a while. Actually there is no evidence that any of the usual treatments seriously increase the risks of an abnormal baby.

It is a sobering thought that 6 per cent of all pregnancies result in some malformation, although, of course, most are trivial. Consequently, on the law of averages, some abnormal babies have been born to mothers taking anti-inflammatory drugs, but there is no evidence that any of them increase this risk. All anti-inflammatory drugs should be avoided in late pregnancy because they increase the chances of maternal and infant haemorrhage, prolong pregnancy and labour and can cause circulatory complications in the new-born.

Of second line drugs, sulphasalazine is safe in pregnancy but chloroquine has caused a few cases of deafness so should be avoided. Gold and penicillamine are not recommended in pregnancy, yet the evidence that they do harm in humans is very slim and many normal babies have been born to women taking these drugs. Many anti-cancer drugs cause foetal damage, yet, curiously, azathioprine does not seem to malform babies and many mothers have had healthy children after taking this drug throughout pregnancy. Steroids in the doses used in arthritis are probably safe. Obviously, we become more aware of drug risks as experience grows but at present any woman who becomes pregnant while on conventional anti-rheumatic drugs should be reassured.

In breast-feeding, chloroquine, gold, penicillamine and immune-suppressants get into the milk and should be avoided. Sulphasalazine, anti-inflammatory drugs and steroids appear to be safe.

11
Alternative Medicine

Alternative medicine is a poor name, implying you must choose between it and conventional medicine, whereas actually they overlap. Many doctors now accept aspects of osteopathy, acupuncture and homeopathy and tolerate the fact that half their patients use patent remedies of no proven value, provided these do not displace adequate conventional treatment and are safe. The practice of surgery and drugs such as gold, once heretical, are now orthodox while time-hallowed conventional treatments continue to be discarded as valueless.

On what basis do we come to accept some unorthodox therapies and reject others? Although we are prejudiced by professional pride we are no more narrow-minded than many alternative practitioners and their clients. Doctors interpret disease with the concepts of modern biological science, so they automatically reject theories expressed in non-physiological mumbo-jumbo. They also mistrust emotional justifications for the value of treatments such as their being 'natural' – tobacco and malaria mosquitoes are natural too. From time to time we have to accept treatments that prove useful but have no rational basis and we then try to explain them in scientifically acceptable terms, as we do with acupuncture, for example.

The main objection to alternative therapies is that with few exceptions there is no reliable information from clinical trials to show that they work. However, most alternative treatments for arthritis claim that they are proven to work, so what is wrong with the proof offered? It relies almost exclusively on anecdotes, often involving testimonials from particular patients, and this is not acceptable evidence. If you had nasty rheumatoid arthritis and someone showed you letters from people he claimed to have cured of arthritis, or photographs of rough arthritic joints that had become smooth, you might be inclined to believe him. But what does he mean by arthritis? Did his patients just have the trivial aches and pains of 'rheumatism' that clear up anyway, or ar arthritis like Reiter's disease, which often only lasts a short time? If some did have rheumatoid, could they have had a natural remission? You are probably unaware that the apparent miracle remodelling of badly damaged joints can also occur naturally. What you need to know is how many people took his treatment, and if the number who responded differed significantly from what would have occurred by chance. Only a controlled trial can tell you that.

Consider also why we bother with dummy tablets in medical trials. Why not give no treatment at all to the control group? If we did this, all treatments would appear to be effective since we know from studies that all conditions respond to dummy treatment better than no treatment at all. Bear this in mind when you hear claims for the more elaborate treatments such as bee-stings and spas where placebo comparison is impossible.

In the absence of trials we cannot know about side-effects either, although where we have tried to find out, adverse reactions seem uncommon. Since I regard most alternative treatments as untried, or shown to be ineffective, I believe you have to accept one inevitable 'side-effect' of taking them – the risk that your disease will run its natural course. Doctors see the tragedies of those patients who, understandably frustrated by slow progress on orthodox treatment, return wrecked after a few years experimenting with fringe cures. Our dislike of alternative therapy is as much for its human consequences as its intellectual dishonesty. The US Consumers' Union has drawn up a list of features that are typical of 'quack' practitioners:

1.   He may offer a special or secret formula for curing arthritis.
2.   He advertises and uses case histories from satisfied patients.
3.   He may promise a quick or easy cure.
4.   He may claim to know the cause of arthritis and may talk about 'cleansing your body of poisons'.
5.   He may say surgery, X-rays and drugs prescribed by a physician are unnecessary.
6.   He may accuse the medical establishment of deliberately blocking progress or of persecuting him.
7.   He does not let his method be tested in tried and proven ways.

DIET

Doctors are thought to have arrogant disregard for the role of diet in arthritis. Certainly I get irritated by the evangelism of the dietary lobby and I reject personal anecdotes that changing the diet can cure arthritis. However, I am happy for my patients to experiment with diet if they want to, and there is a rational explanation of how diet may help.

Complex fatty acids form the starting point for chemical chain reactions that generate many inflammatory mediator substances, including prostaglandins. In animals some inflammatory processes can be modified by altering dietary fatty acid. Some recent, properly conducted, studies show that diets rich in fish oils – 'the eskimo diet' – produce slight benefit in terms of pain and inflammation in rheumatoid arthritis, but they are not 'cures'. As *The Lancet* commented, if they were pills, they would be insufficiently effective to get a product licence. Some bowel diseases have an associated arthritis and subtle changes may be seen in the gut of patients with other arthritic conditions, including rheumatoid arthritis, but their meaning and relation to diet is unclear. Coeliac disease is a bowel disorder due to an allergy to the wheat protein gluten, and a small number of these patients have an arthritis which responds to gluten-free food, but only a handful of people with true rheumatoid type arthritis have been shown to have food allergy. There is nothing in the idea that 'acid foods' are bad for arthritis.

Controlled trials of diet are difficult because you cannot check if the patient is sticking to it and because it is difficult to design a placebo. In addition, experiments show that weight loss itself reduces the intensity of joint inflammation, and most diet treatments are low in calories and produce early weight loss. If you are overweight it is sensible to slim down – at least it takes the strain off your joints. However, most severe rheumatoid patients are skinny and more likely to be undernourished.

Evening Primrose Oil and Cod-liver Oil

You can see from the last section how altering the fatty acids of the body might reduce the severity of inflammatory arthritis, and a recent trial shows that a number of rheumatoid patients taking either evening primrose oil or cod-liver oil could partly reduce their need for anti-inflammatory drugs. We are not talking about a cure, however, and larger studies are still needed.

Seatone

Seatone is a very expensive preparation made from the New Zealand green-lipped mussel which has been widely publicised. Much less well reported is the fact that a controlled trial in the *British Medical Journal* in 1981 showed it to be quite ineffective in the treatment of rheumatoid arthritis. A few minor side-effects were observed.

HERBAL AND SIMILAR REMEDIES

The range of these preparations is enormous. Most are no doubt harmless and those which contain natural aspirin-like substances such as feverfew or willow bark may have a mild anti-inflammatory effect. Virtually none has the backing of controlled studies and the justification for their use is fanciful. Cider vinegar with honey is a popular example – based on the idea that vinegar will dissolve the calcium around stiff joints and that the honey will keep it in solution. Believe it if you must. Royal jelly from the salivary glands of the worker bee has been subject to a proper trial in osteo-arthritis and did not work. To many, the value of these products is that they are 'natural', but beware the hand of man in nature: one patient nearly died after taking an 'ancient Chinese herbal preparation' which had been laced by the manufacturer with modern anti-rheumatic drugs to improve its effects.

OTHER TREATMENTS
Homeopathy

Homeopathy is based on the assumption that symptoms reflect the body's attempt to overcome disease and that natural substances which produce similar symptoms can do good in very dilute amounts. This has a certain logic and homeopathy is now available on the NHS. Homeopaths use several preparations together because they claim to treat the many aspects that make up the whole patient rather than just a disease. *Rhus tox* is widely included for anti-rheumatic properties. There is a trial which shows it to have a slight anti-inflammatory effect in rheumatoid arthritis, and another showing it to be ineffective in osteo-arthritis.

Acupuncture

It is not well known that acupuncture was once commonly used by British doctors and advocated for back pain up to this century. It is interesting that its fall from favour coincided with the discovery of aspirin. There is a large scientific literature on acupuncture and physiological explanations can be offered to explain its action. Currently in favour is the evidence that acupuncture increases the levels of natural morphine-like substances in the brain (endorphins). Acupuncture is not a cure for anything, but there is some support for an effect in back pain similar to that obtained by simple analgesics. Interestingly, tests have shown it does not really matter where the needles are placed. Studies on acupuncture are hard to design fairly and a recent detailed study shows that all seven published trials on acupuncture in rheumatoid arthritis are meaningless.

Osteopathy

This is a technique for manual correction of alleged spinal displacements and some of its techniques are used by physiotherapists and doctors. Many of us do not believe the confident assertions osteopaths make as to the cause of spinal problems but many of us accept that they provide quite rapid relief for a few patients with acute neck or backache. However, controlled trials in large numbers of patients show that, overall, osteopathy is no more beneficial than other treatments or placebo manipulation. I do not believe osteopathy prevents recurrence of spinal pain.

Chiropractic

Chiropractitioners also manipulate the back but use a different technique. They also attribute a much wider range of disorders, diabetes, for example, to spinal derangements, which I find totally absurd. One imperfect study of chiropractic in back pain showed no advantage over the usual treatments.

Copper Bracelets

I see copper bracelets on patients suffering painful conditions ranging from backache to severe rheumatoid arthritis. I hope after reading this book you will agree what a sad reflection it is on our education of the public that they could imagine a single cure for such different disorders. Needless to say, there are no controlled studies of copper bracelets and the same goes for all the myriad other 'cures', from aromatherapy to bee stings.

Index